Fat Loss

The Biology of Weight Control

Ray Reynolds

CONTENTS

1 INTRODUCTION

Although I included a few of my favorite Paleo recipes at the end of this book and a link to my favorite Ketogenic recipe site this is not a Paleo recipe book. It is also not your typical Paleo Diet book; there are literally hundreds of those to choose from. I am a research biologist who has dedicated 40 years of his life to learning how our bodies function. What I have learned is that Mother Nature is very synergistic and has a wicked sense of humor.

I worked on one project for a major pharmaceutical company trying to isolate the chemical in strawberries that prevents the generation of capillaries in tumors. If we had succeeded it would have been worth billions of dollars per year to the company. In the end we spent millions of research dollars engineering an artificial strawberry, which was not patentable because it had every chemical that the strawberry did. Management was not happy! Big Pharma believes more in the efficacy of natural cures than the practitioners of holistic medicine. They try to patent Mother Nature every day. So far with zero success!

If you approach Paleo dieting solely as a short-term fat loss diet you will miss out on 70% of the benefits. The initial fat loss is just the beginning and is somewhat artificial in nature compared to the total health benefits you will experience about three to six months into a continuous Ketogenic diet.

The only reason that a person's body fat percentage is ever higher than 10% in men or 15% in women is that they have type two diabetes, which is caused by the overproduction of insulin. This is the opposite of type one diabetes, which is genetic and caused by a lack of insulin production. The sole purpose of insulin is to transport excess glucose from our blood plasma into our fat cells and store it there for later use as a source of energy when our blood and liver glucose levels become depleted.

Binge eating, metabolic syndrome, fatty liver disease, poor kidney function and many other modern day health problems are cured once this insulin resistance is brought under control. If you are thinking that this book will not help you lose your fat because "you do not have diabetes." please read the following.

The sole function of insulin is to transport blood glucose into your fat cells converting it to lipids along the way. If too much fat is being transported to and stored in your fat cells doesn't it make sense that you have too high a level of insulin? That is after all the only way it can get there. The definition of type two diabetes is "The over production of insulin causing desensitization, which further increases the production of insulin." This causes an ever-escalating cycle of insulin over production and obesity is the end result.

Let me use myself as an example of what you can expect if you are persistent. About five years ago my insulin resistance got to the point that eating one slice of pizza would cause so much over production of insulin that it would transport all of the glucose from my blood into my fat cells. This would happen so fast that my metabolism did not have sufficient time to switch to Ketogenesis and I would pass out. Unlike most people I understood why and immediately started eliminating all carbohydrates from my diet. I also started intermittent fasting. I failed! Carbohydrates are more addictive than heroin. After a few weeks I tried again.

This time I only cut my sugar intake by 50% and continued to eat bread. When I felt that I had finally adjusted to that level of carb intake I made another 50% cut. As we will find out in later chapters the high level of insulin in the absence of glucose causes an artificial and persistent feeling of hunger that will completely disappear once your insulin production is brought under control.

Yesterday I ate breakfast at noon. It consisted of two fried eggs and three strips of bacon. I skipped lunch and that evening I had a piece of lasagna and went to bed. This morning when I got up I walked a mile to the gym and lifted weights for an hour I then walked home showered, changed clothes and then walked three miles to the central market to purchase groceries.

I then arrived back home at 1:00 and was thinking about finally having breakfast when I got distracted by some work I was doing on the computer and forgot to eat. It is currently 6:00 pm and I am still not hungry. I have fasted for 24 hours and still have no interest in food. I am currently at 15% body fat and losing it at an alarming rate. I have more energy than ever because my body is currently in hunting mode the same as our Paleolithic ancestors when they where searching for their next meal.

Under those circumstances suffering from hunger and

having low energy was not a survival trait. When we have normal insulin levels we feel no hunger and actually are much more energetic when in ketosis. I will probably have something to eat prior to going to bed but it would not be because I am hungry and I will make sure that it is 100% protein and fat so that I will continue to burn fat as I sleep.

When I finally reach a 10% body fat level in another month or so my body will start producing enough hunger hormone that I will not be able to reduce my fat level any further. On the other hand I will be able to consume 10,000 calories (as long as none of them are from sugars) per day and not gain fat.

All of the extra calories will be burned off through the production of body heat instead of being stored as fat. This is how a normally regulated metabolism works. This is why your skinny friend can eat as much as she wants and not gain an ounce of fat. Her metabolism is not out of adjustment because of abnormal insulin levels.

More than a third of the American population is currently classified as obese. Let's investigate the cause from the perspective of current scientific research rather than popular opinion. But first it is 7:00 pm and I am finally going to go have breakfast! Won't take long I'll be right back.

Life as it was

Our bodies are designed for life, as it was 100,000 or more years ago. Agriculture had not been invented yet so there was no continuous supply of calories available to keep us going. We were hunter-gatherers who might get lucky and have a surplus of food one day and then none for the next four. To cope with this our bodies had long ago developed the ability to store energy in the form of fat and then utilize that stored energy for fuel when no other food was available.

Carbohydrates in whatever form are first used to make blood glucose. When our bodies have enough to supply our current energy needs, the remainder is turned into fat for future use. There are only two types of sugar that can cross the brain blood barrier and nourish it, Glucose and Ketones. After about 14 hours without carbohydrate consumption our blood glucose levels become low enough that our bodies switch over to converting our fat stores to ketones.

Obviously blood glucose depletion occurred on a regular basis when we were hunter-gatherers. This was not normally a problem since our bodies would simply switch over to converting fat to ketones, which then were used by our bodies for energy until such time as we were able to find a source of carbohydrates and once again increase our blood glucose to a sufficiently high level that it could be used as the primary energy source. If we were lucky we would have enough glucose left over to store some as fat for later use.

In that era our diets mainly consisted of fats and proteins from eating insects and animals. Most of our carbohydrate intake came from seasonal fruits and tubers. Honey, while an obvious and desirable energy source was very dangerous to gather and often proved fatal to the gatherer. Because the consumption of carbohydrates was so necessary for survival and so difficult to obtain, an insatiable appetite for anything sweet was a survival trait and since it was impossible to consume too much carbohydrates because of their limited supply it was a completely unregulated desire.

Much of our physiology is based upon survival during that era. Saber toothed cats and packs of dire wolves were the least of the predatory concerns. The bears were 30% larger than a modern-day brown bear and could run considerably faster.

While monkeys have a very high strength to weight ratio and can climb their way to safety. Our ancestors had to stand their ground and use sharpened poles to persuade apex predators that they were not lunch. Much of our physiology is still based on survival in that harsh environment.

How normal fat storage works

In that era corpulence was not a survival characteristic but staying warm was. They did not call it the "Ice Age" for no reason. A "normally functioning" body has a very tightly regulated fat set point of around 10% of body weight. A healthy 150-pound person will have about 15 pounds of fat stores, which is more than enough to survive for two weeks without food.

If we already had enough fat to be at our "fat set point" any excess calories would immediately be burned off as body heat by increasing the basal metabolic rate as much as 50%. This higher metabolic rate also increased our strength and endurance as well as mental acuity while we were trying to find that next meal, which hopefully would contain enough carbohydrates that we could replenish our dwindling fat stores. All of these biological processes were very tightly controlled by our genetics and required no conscious thought to maintain in equilibrium.

Infants are born with what is called brown fat. Their bodies use it as a catalyst to help burn their white belly fat to generate heat and keep them warm. This brown fat is usually located on our backs and is always present in persons who live in cold climates. Both its' formation and utilization are triggered by our feeling cold.

Because we are so efficient at heating our homes and have very warm clothing to wear almost no one today has any of this type of fat. The only thing that will cause our bodies to form this brown fat is feeling cold. Here in Arequipa, Peru, which is at 8,000' altitude the nighttime temperature is 40-50 degrees but I never feel cold even though I am only wearing a tee shirt. In an unheated house I sleep without a shirt or blanket to keep me warm, under a single cotton sheet and never feel cold. My body burns an enormous amount of fat producing enough body heat so that I do not feel cold.

This is how a well-regulated metabolism was meant to function. Don't make yourself miserable all the time trying to duplicate this until you have regulated the rest of your metabolism but be aware of it and try not to over dress or over heat your house to keep yourself too warm.

As a side note torso fat is always the last to be used by our bodies. They will first use all of the fat from our appendages, including or faces before belly fat. The reason for this is that the fat on our torsos is there to act as insulation to protect our internal organs from the extreme cold. There is no exercise or diet that will specifically target fat deposits in a specific area of the body. It is all controlled by genetics not what we eat or what we do.

There are also deposits of fat surrounding our internal organs inside our abdominal cavities. This type of fat is very difficult to eliminate and is what causes a "Pot Belly". Unfortunately this is the last type of fat to be burned by our bodies and usually only after the external subcutaneous fat has been exhausted.

Our fat set point made sure that we always had sufficient fat stores to survive until the next meal. At the same time it also made sure that we were sufficiently lean and fast to chase down and catch a rabbit. Carbohydrates were very important for survival. If we found any fruit trees or other sources of concentrated carbohydrates we would camp there and consume as much as we could over several days until there was none left and we had stored as much fat as possible. It was an insatiable desire for the sweet taste of those apples or berries that motivated us not reason or understanding of biology. Survival characteristics only work if they are hard wired into every fiber of our being and this all worked perfectly until the modern era.

Today we use fewer calories to maintain our bodies because of our easier workloads but at the same time we have readily available sources of cheap high glycemic food to store as fat. This makes our bodies very happy because they have an endless supply of carbohydrates to convert into fat for the future famine, which never comes. We have so lost touch with reality that we think that being in ketosis is a bad thing that can be solved by simply eating something. In reality having low blood glucose and using our fat stores for energy is historically our normal state and not something to be avoided.

The Modern history of dieting

It was 1861 and Dr. William Banting of London, England had a problem. At over 200 pounds he was seriously over weight and wanted to lose as much fat as possible. He consulted with some of his fellow physicians who suggested that he needed more exercise so he decided to take up rowing on the local river. He wasn't able to lose any weight but he did work up a very healthy appetite! He consulted with some other physicians who recommended that he decrease his caloric intake, which he did. He didn't lose any weight but was always tired, cold and hungry.

Eventually his problem came to the attention of a French

physician who recommended a special diet consisting of meat and fish with green vegetables. No carbohydrates were allowed. Over the following year he lost his fat and was so pleased with the results that he published a pamphlet describing this diet entitled "Letter on Corpulence" which in 1863 became the first diet book ever published. So the Ketogenic diet has been used for at least 150 years.

A few years later Dr. William Osler who wrote "The Principles and Practices of Medicine" and is considered to be the father of modern medicine, published his own book espousing the benefits of the high fat low carb diet for weight lose. Today everyone thinks that the Paleo or Ketogenic diet is a modern discovery when in reality it has been popular for more than 150 years.

By the 1950s this concept of using a low carb high fat diet to lose weight was very popular and everyone knew that it was white carbohydrates and especially starchy foods and sugar that caused people to gain weight.

In the 1960s we became more sedentary and the incidence of heart disease began to increase. Fat was thought to be the culprit because it tended to raise LDL cholesterol, which was perceived by the American Medical Association as being the cause of coronary artery blockage. The result was that by the 1970s high fat low carb diets were being vilified as unhealthy fads that were causing the increase in coronary disease. The problem with this approach was that if you could not consume a diet that was rich in fats and proteins you had to switch to one that was high in carbohydrates.

Unfortunately fattening carbohydrates could not be substituted as they were what caused obesity. The AMA's solution to this cognitive dissonance was to promote "healthy" whole grains as the carbohydrates of choice. It was easy to convince the public that fat was what made people fat. It sounded so logical. How could "Fat" not make you fat? It was after all "FAT". The "fattening carbohydrates" model of fat production became the "Calories in - Calories out" model that we are so familiar with today. This erroneous concept that eating fat is what causes fat to be stored on our bodies still persists to this day and is one of the many reasons that people fail to control their body fat levels.

There was still much debate between the dietary fats and dietary carbs proponents, which was resolved in 1977 not by scientific research but by government fiat. The USDA declared that Americans could greatly improve their health and reduce their probability of heart attacks by reducing the amount of fats in their diet.

Nutrition had moved from the arena of scientific research and discovery to being a political football. A few incompetent thinkers backed up by the government completely altered the eating habits of Americans. None of this was backed up by direct scientific research or even empirical analysis. It was all based on hubris, ego and supposition. In a relatively short time Americans transitioned from a high fat diet to one that consisted of 60% carbohydrates.

This was the origin of the food pyramid, which has meat at the apex to be eaten once a week or even monthly with pasta, grains, bread and rice forming the base and being consumed daily. The only good part was that exercise was considered very important. By 1995 The American Heart Association was recommending that to control the amount of fat and cholesterol it was better to eat "low fat cookies or crackers, unsalted pretzels, candy, gum drops and sugary syrups."

So the message from the medical establishment became very clear. You could eat any amount of fattening carbohydrates that you wanted to as long as you avoided fats. People for some strange reason tend to perceive governmental advice as accurate so unfortunately compliance to these guidelines was enthusiastic. We ate less eggs and meat resulting in a reduction of fat consumption from 45% to 35% of total dietary calories. At the same time we were exercising more and dramatically reducing the percentage of citizens who smoked. This had a very positive effect on heart health. The incidence of hypertension was reduced by 40% as well as reducing cholesterol levels by 28%.

Unfortunately the increased consumption of carbohydrates was having its' effect as well. Not only did our consumption of grains and starchy vegetables increase dramatically but also the consumption of sugar. During the 1800s the per capita consumption of sugar was about 5 pounds per year. As the sugar cane production in the Caribbean and southern portion of the US increased so did the availability of cheap sugar.

By 2013 the per capita consumption of sugar had increased to more than 110 pounds per year. So from the 1960s to today we experienced an unprecedented shift in our eating habits from a very high percentage of fat consumption to carbohydrates and more importantly to refined white sugar.

As with most everything we consume our taste receptors build up a tolerance for sweetness over time with the result that we require an ever increasing amount of sugar to stimulate the same sensation of sweetness. As a result of this, other healthy naturally sweet foods such as vegetables no longer taste sweet. This creates a very unnatural physiological demand on the part of our bodies for an ever-increasing amount of sugar intake. Producers of processed foods were very quick to realize this and as a result kept raising the amount of sugar in their products to keep up with this increase in tolerance for sweetness on the part of their customers.

In 1950 the per capita consumption of wheat was 125 pounds per year by 2002 it had reached 150 pounds per year. The tipping point was 1977 with the release of the first dietary guidelines for Americans. From that point on the incidence of obesity steadily increased. The reason that we do not actually think about the causes of obesity is that we think that we already know what causes it.

Changes in US food consumption 1970 to 2013

Butter	-40%
Eggs	-20%
Meat	-15%
Grains	+40%
Sugar	+200%

Annual sugar consumption - pounds per capita

1800	5 pounds
1820	7 pounds
1840	10 pounds
1860	25pounds
1880	30pounds
1900	45pounds

1920	65pounds
1940	80pounds
1960	80pounds
1980	85pounds
2014	120pounds

Pounds of yearly grain consumption per capita

Grain	1950s	1960s	1970s	1980s	1990s	2000
Wheat	126	115	113	122	142	146
Corn	15	13	11	17	24	29
Rice	5	7	8	12	18	29
Total	146	135	134	151	184	204

Obesity as a percentage of population

	1977	1990	2005
Overweight	31%	32%	35%
Obese	15%	23%	35%
Very Obese	2%	3%	5%

2 CALORIES IN - CALORIES OUT

This is the famous calories in calories out model of weight control, which has been en vogue since the 1970s. It basically states that if your fat percentage is increasing it is because you are either eating too much or exercising too little. This reduces fat control to personnel choices. If you are fat it is because you are either a sloth or a glutton or both and ignores the more nuanced possibilities.

One of the hallmarks of this theory is that a calorie of fat is no different than a calorie of sugar. It states that fat storage is unregulated and that our fat cells are a dump for excess calories of any type or quantity. It also states that this process is under conscious control. All of these suppositions completely ignore the effects of hunger and basal metabolic rate.

Another assumption is that the intake and expenditure of calories are independent of each other. In other words eating too much has no impact on the amount of exercise you do and likewise exercise does not affect what and how much you eat. Technically overeating with no corresponding increase in exercise will promote weight gain.

If you have ever been in an airport during a major holiday you might assume that too many people coming into the airport and too few leaving cause the crowding. That information while true is not as useful as you might think. The real reason is that it is a major holiday so the airport has more passengers than is usual. The same is true for calories. What is driving them in and what is keeping them from leaving is the way that the question needs to be phrased if we are to arrive at a usable answer.

The reason that most people believe that weight gain is a behavioral problem is that it is so simple, logical and obvious. It appeals to our sense of self-determinism and makes us feel in control of our destinies. Without the necessary understanding of the biology involved it is impossible to understand how truly complex the process is. The proponents of the calorie in calorie out model of weight control consider weight control as more of a psychological problem than a physiological one.

When the results of their experiments do not produce lasting weight loss it always comes down to whether the persons involved were gluttons or sloths. Defects in character are always easier to blame for poor research results than the theories themselves. Perhaps the researchers should have considered their own lack of objectivity instead.

Much of our knowledge of biology is based on empirical observation and supposition rather than a detailed working knowledge of how a very complex biochemical process actually works. The calorie in calorie out model of weight loss has been tested for decades with very poor results but still it persists and is still the go to method for attempts at fat loss.

Why calorie restricted diets do not work

In 1917 the Carnegie Institute of Nutrition conducted a study of 12 Young men who were placed on a very low calorie diet of 1400 - 2000 calories per day. The subjects continually complained about how hungry they were and found it nearly impossible to keep warm no matter how much clothing they wore. When the researchers investigated these complaints they discovered that their base metabolic rate had decreased by more than 30%. Immediately after the experiment the subjects over ate and immediately regained any fat that they had lost.

In 1944 the University of Minnesota conducted a more extensive study of 36 men who were placed on a six month 1600 calorie per day diet. Within a week their basal metabolic rate dropped by 40% and heart volume by 20% their body temperatures were also lower. When they finished the study they immediately started binge eating. This increased appetite continued for as much as one year after the study was terminated. There was a residual effect and this is true of either extreme. If people are forced to appreciably reduce their daily caloric intake for a period of time they inevitably over eat for an even longer period of time.

In a more recent 1995 study by Dr. Rudolph Leibel that was reported in the New England Journal of Medicine 18 obese and 23 non-obese participants we're fed a standardized meal so that all of them were sure to receive precisely the same amount of calories per day. It was determined that when their caloric intake was increased sufficiently to produce a 10% increase in body fat their metabolic rates would increase by at least 15% and most of the additional calories that were being consumed we're simply burned off as body heat.

Research studies that place people on very low calorie diets for extended periods were shown to cause minor weight loss but the participants always complained of being cold and lethargic. This was caused by a very significant 30-40% decrease in their basal metabolic rates. Their bodies were limiting the use of calories for heat production. Heart rate and blood pressure also decreased and their bodies exhibited all of the symptoms of shutting down to conserve energy. These early studies also demonstrated that after resuming a normal diet our bodies tend to maintain a slower metabolic rate for an extended period allowing the body to use the greater number of calories available to add more fat than when they started the diet.

When caloric intake is low our metabolisms slow down to compensate. The opposite is true as well. When caloric intake is higher than needed the normal response is to burn off the calories, usually in the form of body heat rather than store them. A person with normal insulin production whose body is functioning correctly will not store every surplus calorie as fat. This will only happen when our bodies feel that our fat storage is too low for survival purposes.

It appears that one of the key assumptions of the calories in calories out model of weight control is incorrect. Caloric intake and expenditure are very closely linked and codependent. If we increase our caloric intake our metabolisms tend to increase and burn off the excess calories. When our caloric intake is reduced our bodies tend to conserve caloric usage by reducing our basal metabolic rate. This point of equilibrium is referred to as our metabolic set point and is determined by genetics and hormonal secretion.

A normally functioning body will try to maintain its' body fat percentage at about 10%. All research studies both past and recent indicate that our bodies will adjust our basal energy expenditure to burn off excess calories and will then reduce our energy expenditure whenever our caloric intake is reduced.

When the study participants' caloric intake was returned to

normal and they lost the 10% extra fat that they had gained they actually experienced a slight reduction in their original fat levels because their basal metabolic rates were slightly higher than before beginning the weight increase. So it would appear that it might actually be more beneficial to increase caloric consumption for a short period of time so that when you return to your normal eating habits your body will naturally consume fewer calories and therefore produce a slight fat loss. (NEJM 1995 march 9, 332 (10); 621-28)

Yet another study reported in the American Journal of clinical nutrition in 2008 demonstrated that after the participants had maintained a 10% weight loss during the study their basil metabolic rate remained as much as 10% lower for an additional year. (Am J Clin Nutr 2008; 88; 906-912)

A study reported in the 2011 edition of the New England Journal of Medicine demonstrates why this happens. Whenever a person experiences fat loss there is a proportionate long term increase in the hormone that causes us to feel hungry (ghrelin) and a decrease in the hormones that reduce our feelings of hunger. The opposite is also true. Whenever we increase our consumption of food and consequently our fat level the level of hunger hormone is decreased and the levels of the other hormones that control hunger are increased so that we lose our appetite and our fat level returns to its normal set point. (N Engl J Med 2011;365:1597-1604)

In a normal body a 10% increase in caloric intake will cause a 15% increase in energy expenditure whereas a 10% decrease in caloric intake will cause a 15% decrease in energy expenditure. This condition persists for as much as a year after your fat level returns to its former set point. If our bodies are functioning properly their body fat percentage is very closely regulated at a set point of about 10% of body weight for men and 15% for women.

Now let's take a look at the largest research study of the calorie in calorie out model ever attempted "The 1993 Women's Health Initiative Dietary Modification Trial". This was an eight-year dietary study of 50,000 women. They were divided into two groups one allowed to eat whatever they normally did and a second group that was given a diet high in vegetables and fiber.

For seven years the caloric intake of the second group was maintained at 1800 calories per day, which was about 400 calories less then what was necessary to maintain their basil metabolic rate. They also exercised an extra 10% per day. The end result after 7 to 9 years of continuous effort was that the low caloric intake group lost less then one kilo of weight per participant compared to the control group who did nothing.

Are you beginning to understand why it's so difficult for you to lose your fat by calorie restriction? Unfortunately it gets worse. Half of their weight loss was lean body mass not fat and their average waist circumference increased by half an inch! A pound of fat contains 3000 calories. If they were running a 400-calorie per day deficit they should have lost at least one pound of fat every ten days or three pounds per month. That would add up to 36 pounds for the first year.

When you try to reduce your caloric intake to lose fat it sets up a vicious cycle of energy conservation and increased hunger hormone production, which will bring you right back to your original set point. The first rule of fat reduction is do not artificially restrict your caloric intake. Calorie restricted diets have a perfect forty year track record unblemished by success!

What happens is when you begin your calorie reduction diet and reduce your caloric intake by 10% your body will reduce its' energy expenditure by 15% to compensate. It will also increase ghrelin production to stimulate your hunger. So you grit your teeth and lose a couple of pounds but then regain a bit because of the decrease in your body's basal metabolic rate.

So to compensate you double down with an exercise program and further calorie restriction, which puts your poor body into panic mode because it assumes that you're too stupid to know that you're hungry and it will increase the production of ghrelin to get the message through to you. If that doesn't work it will assume that no food is available for you to eat.

It then initiates plan B and reduces your basal metabolic rate even more to conserve energy. Eventually this cycle becomes completely intolerable and you give up. The real problem that most people have with fat loss is that to achieve success you have to be smarter than your body and I can assure you that it has a 1 million year head start on the fat manipulation learning curve.

If you really believe that eating too much is what causes you to be fat that hypothesis is easily tested and has been on numerous occasions since the 1960s. Ethan Sims was an endocrinologist who conducted a study of overeating on convicts in the Vermont state prison. He fed them anywhere from 4,000 to 10,000 calories per day. Initially their weight went up slightly but after a relatively short period of time it would stabilize and their basal metabolic rates were proven to be 50% greater than normal. Their bodies were simply burning off the excess calories as body heat.

Another large seven-year study was conducted in 2010. 40,000 women were divided into three groups the first group exercised for one hour per week; the second group did seven hours of exercise per week and a third group exercised two hours per day. At the end of the seven-year study there was almost no difference in weight gain or loss amongst the three different exercise groups. (jama 2010, 303 (12)

1173-1179 Busing et all)

Another similar study in 2007 used a group of 100 men and 100 women the entire group performing six hours of exercise per week for one year. The entire study group had been very sedentary previously so they were basically going from zero exercise to at least one hour of aerobic exercise per day. By the end of the one-year study the women had lost three pounds of fat and men four pounds. So once again extreme exercise does not seem to increase fat loss very much. (Mactiernan et all Obesity (2007) 15, 1496-1512)

Another research group in Denmark decided that if a little exercise is good for you then lots of exercise must be better so they trained a group of sedentary people to run a marathon! The men in the group lost an average of five pounds and the women experienced no change in fat to muscle ratio. This indicates that there was no appreciable gaining of muscle weight that offset any loss of fat.

Our bodies have a hormonally controlled compensatory mechanism that acts much as a thermostat does to regulate a room's temperature. This regulation of fat level tends to overcompensate. When we are deprived of calories our bodies produce the hormone ghrelin, which increases our appetite. Research indicates that this overproduction of the hunger hormone persists for as much as a year after our fat level returns to normal. The same studies indicated that the hormones that tell your body that you're full are produced at a lower level than before the attempted weight loss.

So it is very possible that dieting even on a small scale can actually produce a weight gain instead of weight loss overtime. What our bodies are attempting to do here is keep us from starving to death. Remember that our physiology was designed for life in the Paleolithic when the odds of us gaining too much fat were zero but there was a very high probability that we would starve to death or be eaten by a predator if we did not have enough energy to run fast.

It was a perpetual biological balancing act of having sufficient fat stores that we would not starve and maintaining a strength to weight ratio that would allow us to either fight or flee a predator. Our genetics are still the same and our bodies are obsessed with conserving energy expenditure because it has always been a viable survival strategy.

These results have been the same throughout all the major studies conducted to determine whether exercise contributes to fat loss. Exercise is very beneficial for your health. It is a major factor in preventing both cancer and heart disease. To my knowledge there has never been a study that has successfully linked fat loss to exercise. The reasons for this is that no matter how hard you try to maintain a steady intake of calories throughout such a program your real intake will increase slightly as your body compensates for the added calorie expenditures provided by the exercise.

Our bodies are extremely efficient so the amount of calories that are burned in one hour of exercising are so small that it only requires an equally small increase in caloric intake to offset it. The other reason that it doesn't work is that when we elect to exercise on a regular basis throughout the week we are too tired to perform other spontaneous activities during our daily lives that we usually do that would burn calories. This is referred to as compensation.

Another thing that people do not understand is that the vast majority of the calories that we consume each day are used to maintain our basal metabolic rate. The basal metabolic rate for a 140-pound person is 2,200 calories. Every single one of those 2,200 calories is used in one day even if you perform no physical activity at all. You will only burn 100 calories during a brisk 45-minute walk. Studies have proven that no matter how vigorously a person exercises it only accounts for approximately 5% of their daily caloric intake. Most of our caloric expenditure every day is used just to heat our bodies.

It is very easy for bodies to compensate for the 5% extra caloric usage caused by exercising by simply reducing our metabolic rate and cutting back on the heating. The real benefits of exercising daily are very real but fat loss is not one of them. It is obvious that the "Calorie in Calorie out" hypothesis of fat control does not work.

Now the fun starts. First everyone blames the victims telling them they didn't have enough willpower and that they were cheating on their diet. This type of abuse isn't restricted to your mother-in-law. Health professionals are guilty of the same sin. But what is infinitely more damaging is when the victim starts blaming themselves for their failure.

3 THE HORMONAL HYPOTHESIS

According to this theory your level of insulin is what determines your fat storage set point and the amount of fat that will be transported into your fat cells. This seems to make sense because there is no bodily function that is not very tightly regulated by our hormones.

A research study conducted in 2001 divided a group of type one diabetics into two groups one of which used a greater number of insulin injections to tightly control their condition. The second group's injection rate was much more loosely controlled. What the researchers found in the first group was that the greater amount of insulin that was being injected caused major weight gain in 30% of the test subjects. There was a very strong and direct correlation between the quantity of insulin that was injected and the amount of fat the subjects gained during the study. (Diabetes Care 2001, 24: 1711-1722)

What they discovered was very interesting. When the participants began the study they were consuming 2000 calories per day with no increase in fat percentage. By the end of the study they were only consuming 1700 calories per day but had still managed to gain an average of 20 pounds of extra fat per participant.

Another study that was reported in the British medical journal "The Lancet" showed that whenever you increase the quantity of insulin therapy received by type 2 diabetics there is always a corresponding increase in their fat level. (The Lancet, vol. 352, 1998, pp. 837-853) In actual fact you can produce a corresponding proportional weight gain in non-diabetics by injecting them with insulin.

Another study that was recorded in the New England Journal of Medicine in 2007 demonstrated the same correlation between the amount of insulin that diabetics received and the amount of fat gain they experienced. (N Engl J Med 2007;357:1716-30 Holman RR)

There is also a common localized condition called insulin Lipohypertrophy. This causes fat deposits to occur surrounding areas of the abdomen in which insulin is being injected.

Diabetics often use a drug called Metformin, which does not increase the amount of insulin in their systems but instead directly controls their systemic sugars. When type 2 diabetics reduce their insulin and start relying more on metformin to control their blood sugar they have a corresponding loss of body fat. Another drug called Gliburide is often used to control diabetes and works by increasing the amount of natural insulin production. It also causes a corresponding increase in body fat levels.

From this it is fairly obvious that actual fat gain is very dependent on both blood glucose levels as well as the presence of high levels of insulin. Januvia another type of drug that doesn't raise the insulin levels not only does not cause fat levels to increase it actually causes them to decrease. The same is true of Dapagliflozin, which causes fat loss because it directly reduces blood sugar and does not increase the level of insulin production.

Before insulin therapy was available for the treatment of diabetes a condition known as diabulimia was the result. The lack of sufficient systemic insulin caused type one diabetics to lose all of their body fat no matter how much food they consumed. It is well known within the modern diabetic community that if they want to lose body fat all they need to do is under dose their insulin.

If you administer cortisol to normal people they will gain fat. This is also true of any medical steroids such as prednisone. The overproduction of cortisol is called Cushing's disease. The main symptom is an increase in body fat. The opposite condition or a lack of sufficient cortisol is Addison's disease and its' primary symptom is extreme fat loss. All of this makes it very obvious that the true cause of fat gain and fat loss is not caloric intake per se but hormonal levels. It seems obvious that fat gain or loss is actually controlled more by our insulin and cortisol levels rather than by caloric intake.

Unfortunately the predominant theory of caloric intake versus exercise has caused the so-called experts to focus on behavioral and psychological causes such as fast food, sugar consumption and lack of willpower on the part of the participants rather than the hormonal imbalances that actually promote fat gain or loss.

By taking proactive control of our insulin and cortisol levels we can very quickly eliminate fat from our bodies. You're not becoming fat because you're over eating you're actually over eating because you're getting fat. Now that we understand the root cause of obesity we can start to treat it. It is not predominately a question of caloric intake but a question of what is driving your insulin levels. The answer of course is any food that causes the release of high levels of insulin. This unfortunately includes just about every food that is produced commercially.

That other fat producing hormone cortisol is released when we are under stress. Normally cortisol is only released when we are frightened or upset. It is commonly referred to as the fight or flight hormone. One of its' functions is to shut down any of our systemic processes that it considers to be unnecessary so that our bodies can utilize all of their energy for either fighting the danger or running away from it.

This worked very well for our ancestors during the Paleolithic era but it causes nothing but problems for us today. The reason is that the stress of modern everyday life tends to create a continuous steady drip of cortisol into our system. This impairs the function of our immune systems and also causes our bodies to gain fat the same as insulin.

So in the end the hunger hormones tend to control our fat level set point much as a thermostat would do. We need to examine what and how we eat to determine what is causing our fat level thermostat to malfunction and what we can do to recalibrated it so that it functions properly.

4 THE CAUSES OF INSULIN RESISTANCE

From what we have learned in the preceding chapter it's fairly easy to jump to the conclusion that what abnormally raises our insulin level is the consumption of high glycemic index carbohydrates such as grains, white starchy vegetables and sugars. This is only partially true. Carbohydrate consumption is 15% higher in China and Japan than in the US because rice is a large part of their diets but they have a much lower rate of obesity than in the west. They do however consume 60% less sugar so that their main sources of carbs are medium or low glycemic ones. This lack of excess body fat is not caused by genetic differences. When they move to the US they have the same problem with fat gain that we do.

The cause of insulin resistance

Our bodies tend to moderate and average out the effects that both drugs and hormones have on our bodies. We usually require steadily increasing dosages of most medications to provide the same amount of stimulation as the beginning dosages. This is also true of insulin. Persistent high levels of insulin will cause our bodies to down regulate the receptors that allow it to move glucose out of our blood and into our fat cells. This in turn causes our bodies to respond with ever increasing quantities of insulin to produce the same results as before.

These higher levels of insulin then cause further down regulation of the cell receptors further inhibiting the transport of glucose into our cells. The cycle continues and is self-perpetuating. In order for this cycle to occur a continuously increasing level of insulin must be present in our blood plasma. Periodic high levels of insulin or persistent low-level's will not cause insulin resistance. Both must be present at the same time. This is actually a protective mechanism. If your insulin level was allowed to climb to a high level and remain there for an extended period of time with no decrease in the insulin's effect your blood glucose would drop to 1% or less and you would die.

Insulin Resistance, Ketogenesis and Intermittent Fasting

In the introduction to this book I described how the diet of our ancestors during the Paleolithic era consisted mainly of fats and proteins and how it was very low in carbohydrates and included almost no sugar.

One of the most popular diets for fat loss and control for the last five years has been what is called the Ketogenic or Paleo diet. This is the only form of diet that really works for the elimination of body fat. Weight reduction from every other form of diet is most often caused by short-term water loss or it is some variation of the Ketogenic diet.

A good example of this would be the avocado diet. This one is guaranteed to produce a one-pound fat loss per day. The reason it works is that avocados are almost 100% fat. The only problem with this particular diet is that after twelve days of consuming nothing but avocados you will never be able to eat another one as long as you live!

Then there is the fried pork rind diet. Only eat chicharrónes and the same thing will happen. You will lose about one pound per day of fat without exercising or how about the gallon bucket of lard diet. Same thing, you'll use up all of your blood glucose and go into ketosis. Your body will start breaking down the fat in your fat cells turning it into ketones, which will provide your energy needs. While it is extremely effective for reducing and preventing body fat accumulation most people who use a Ketogenic/Paleo type diet do not understand how it accomplishes this or how to maximize its effectiveness.

The easiest and quickest way to reduce and then eliminate insulin resistance is to eliminate our bodies need for insulin. Since the main reason for the existence of insulin is the transportation of excess glucose from our blood plasma into our fat cells all we need to do is eliminate glucose from our blood plasma and that will eliminate the primary need for insulin production. This is what a Ketogenic diet does.

As was previously stated there are two components involved in causing our bodies to develop a resistance to insulin. They are high systemic levels of insulin and the persistence of those high levels over time. If our breakfast consists of three eggs, four slices of bacon and a slice of toast with butter the only carbohydrates that might increase our insulin level would be the twenty grams from the slice of toast. The remainder of that breakfast is fat or protein, which will have close to zero effect on insulin production.

If you ate dinner at seven o'clock on the previous night and are having your breakfast at seven o'clock the next morning then you have not eaten for twelve hours. This means that your blood glucose level is quite low and as a result the twenty grams of carbohydrates that you just consumed will probably not trigger appreciable increases in your insulin production because your body will need to utilize it immediately for energy.

If however we add in a couple of glasses of orange juice, an extra slice of toast, and jelly as well, that will probably raise our glucose levels to the point where sufficient insulin will need to be produced to move some of that glucose into our fat cells for storage. A very necessary component for the control of insulin production is being in a semi-fasted state for more than twelve hours per 24 hour day.

This is not really difficult to do since we have already fasted for twelve hours from dinner to breakfast. Since all of the glucose produced by any meal will be utilized within three hours of its consumption there will then be an additional three to five semi-fasted hours prior to the next meal. All of this provides us enough time without insulin production so that our bodies do not become resistant to it.

As a side note the consumption of at least thirty grams of protein for breakfast within forty minutes of getting up in the morning will suppress the production of the hunger hormone for the remainder of the morning prior to finally feeling hungry enough to have lunch at one or two o'clock in the afternoon. This is one of the reasons why meals should not be eaten on a ridged schedule. A more natural approach would be to only eat when you really feel hunger.

On the other hand waiting until you are too hungry will cause you to over eat. If too large a portion of that meal is carbohydrate then the blood glucose they produce will be high enough to trigger insulin production, which will then move that glucose into your fat cells for storage. If you could balance your intake of carbs so that they only produce the precise amount of blood glucose that your body currently needs then there would be no excess glucose and therefore no insulin production.

A major contributor to type two diabetes and insulin resistance is continuous snacking on high carb foods throughout the day. This is especially true for children. If you maintain a continuous high-level of insulin for as little as forty hours you will start to develop insulin resistance. It happens very quickly. This new high level of insulin will cause down regulation of the insulin receptors increasing your insulin resistance, which will cause the production of a higher level of insulin to compensate, which will further down regulate the receptors causing further increases in the amount of insulin produced in order to move the excess glucose into your fat cells. Eventually this cycle divorces itself from high glycemic foods and becomes self-perpetuating and independent of the foods that you eat.

In order to start losing fat this cycle must be broken. The only way that this can be accomplished is to eliminate glucose from your blood plasma so that there is no stimulus for the production of insulin. If there is no insulin present for an extended period of time then the insulin receptors, which have been down regulated will respond by up regulating themselves providing the proper level of sensitivity on the occasions when insulin is truly needed to help handle excess blood glucose.

High insulin production causes ever-increasing levels of insulin resistance. High insulin resistance causes high levels of insulin to be produced. It starts out with higher insulin secretion caused by over consumption of high glycemic carbs. If meals or snacks are too close together this then provides the extended period of high insulin necessary to produce type two diabetes. The good news is that since the problem is caused by over production of insulin instead of under production, as is the case with type one diabetes, all you need to do is lower that production for long enough that your insulin receptors normalize.

In a 2009 study of mice with type one diabetes it was shown that the insulin injections that were used to control their condition contributed more to their insulin resistance than their hyperglycemia itself. (J Biol Chem. 2009 October 2; 284(40): 27090-27100, Liu HY)

It has repeatedly been shown that type two diabetes can be induced in healthy persons by injecting them with ever-higher doses of insulin even when their blood glucose is maintained at a normal level. It is the insulin level not the glucose level that causes type two diabetes. (Diabetologia Oct 1994, Vol37, Iss 10, 1025-1035 Del Prato S) (Diabetologia 28:70-75, 1985 Rizza R A)

One study in particular showed that over a six-month study the gradual increase of insulin injection to 100 units per day produced an average gain of 20 pounds in the participants even though their blood glucose levels were always perfect. Their insulin disposal rates which is a measure of how effectively a person utilizes their insulin became progressively worse requiring the ever increasing doses to maintain their glucose levels.

Insulin makes the glucose levels better but the type two diabetes progressively worse. The daily caloric intake of the subjects over the six months dropped from 2000 to 1700 calories but they were still gaining fat. The ever-increasing systemic level of insulin drove this fat gain. When the researchers stopped injecting the insulin the study participants returned to normal and eventually lost their excess fat. This proves that you can produce type two diabetes in healthy people causing them to gain 20 pounds of fat in six months and then return them to normal within a year depending on how much insulin you inject.

Diabetes is driven by insulin over production and the subsequent insulin resistance that results. The way to cure type two diabetes is to limit your glucose level so that it does not trigger the production of insulin. A high fat/low carb diet is simply the easiest way to accomplish this. (Diabetes Care 1993 16: 23-31 Henry R)

Consumption of high glycemic foods is only half of the problem. The other half is that since 1977 there has been a steady increase in the number of times that we eat each day. Instead of three meals per day we consume six, three meals and three snacks. This provides the second part of the insulin resistance equation, an extended period of insulin elevation. (Am J Clin Nutr 2010,91:1342-7 Popkin BM)

Hormones are always released in a pulsatile manner never in a steady stream. When we continually eat and never allow our blood glucose to fall we are creating a very artificial situation that does not occur naturally.

We have gone from the Paleolithic model of extended forced fasting, while we searched desperately for the next meal, which was always very low glycemic, to endlessly grazing like cattle on very high glycemic foods. This is especially prevalent in children and when they establish insulin resistance in their youth it tends to persist into adulthood. Unless that adult makes a conscious effort to understand and cure their problem it will become an ongoing issue. Unlike type one diabetes it will not kill you directly or immediately. It just makes your life miserable to live and creates systemic diseases such as metabolic syndrome and obesity, which eventually will kill you.

Instead of your day being divided between 50% fed and 50% fasted periods of time. It is now more like 70% fed and only 30% fasted. The solution is to go back to restricting your food consumption to an eight to twelve hour time period within each day. The word breakfast was originally two words "break fast". Quite often people would not have dinner and fast from lunch through to their morning meal when they would "break their fast".

Get up early enough each morning so that there is plenty of time to build and eat a proper breakfast or skip it entirely and have an early lunch. What you do not want to do is grab a couple of pop tarts and head to work. That slug of sugar will go straight to your belly.

Most diet books tell you what to eat. The better question is when and what not to eat. It is amazing how little food we need to survive. Once you have cured your insulin resistance and are no longer hungry why eat a large amount of food when you will only burn off those extra calories as heat. Saves a lot on groceries!

The rate of obesity in newborns has tripled since 1980 this is being caused by elevated insulin levels in their mothers. The net result of this is the children are being born fatter then anytime previously. It is obvious that a fetus cannot over eat or under exercise as they have no control over either. This fetal exposure to maternal high levels of insulin gives them a head start on developing their own insulin resistance and obesity after they are born.

We are literally marinating our children in insulin. Their levels are very high prior to their birth and this is setting them up for childhood obesity as they continue to consume high glycemic foods at greater and greater frequencies and quantities every day. Remember that the severity of insulin resistance is time dependent. Also when and how often you eat is just as important as what.

Genetics is a contributor to obesity as well. In studies of adopted children inevitably if the birth parents were fat then the children are as well, regardless of how skinny the adoptive parents are and how conscientious they are of what they feed their adopted children. Studies that have been done of identical twins that were adopted by different families show that both of them have the same phenotype as their birth parents regardless of how they were fed by their adoptive families. Their environment did not influence their corpulence as much as you would expect. Since there is no genetic link that causes over eating or under exercising that is probably not contributing to the problem.

There are people who are genetically more sensitive to insulin and will have higher fat set points because of that but they can still eliminate the excess fat by simply being more proactive about reducing the habits that contribute to their insulin resistance. (Strunkard A J N Engl J Med 1986;314:193-198) (N Engl J Med 1990;322:1483-1487).

In a study of weight gain in the children of diabetics it was found that their genetically set level of insulin sensitivity varied greatly and was determined by how much insulin they secreted in response to a set level of stimulus. So a person's response to a set amount of carbohydrate can be vastly different depending on their genetic sensitivity to them. This response includes both the amount of insulin that is secreted in response to a set amount of carbs as well as the time span of insulin release. (Diabetes 46:1029 1997 Sigal R J) (N engl J Med 2012;367:1387-1396)

There is a common mutation of the insulin sensitivity gene, which causes obesity due to heightened insulin sensitivity. This mutation also contributes to the formation of cancer. This is one of the reasons that obesity has been linked to higher cancer rates. (N engl J Med 2012; 367(11):1002-1011)

Childhood obesity (6-18 year olds) has nearly tripled from 1980 when the low fat high carb dietary model was implemented. These children are not necessarily eating more and exercising less. They have high levels of insulin production, which causes them to become more insulin resistant at a much younger age.

The Pima Indians are the fattest people in the US. They were originally one of the skinniest. Between 1920-1950 they opened trading posts on their reservations where they could purchase nontraditional processed foods. Today their obesity and diabetes rates are more than 50%.

Sumo wrestlers spend a lot of time trying to gain weight. They are very successful at this so if we do the opposite then logically we should loose fat. As it turns out the sumo and average American diet are very similar. They drink a lot of beer, eat large amounts of carbohydrates and sleep after meals. The food they eat is very high carb and low fat. It is obvious that they must be insulin resistant to succeed at gaining so much fat. The reason they eat so much at night is to prevent the fasted period and maintain perpetually high levels of insulin.

Another interesting player in obesity is diet soft drinks that are artificially sweetened. Both the American Heart Association and the American Diabetic Association endorse their consumption and that consumption has tripled since 1977. You would think that this would have some effect on the rate of diabetes but it hasn't. Drinking artificially sweetened beverages actually increases the risk of obesity by 40%. Another study showed a 45% increased risk of Coronary events (Obesity 2008 16:8, 1894-1900, Fowler) and (Journal of General Internal Medicine 2012 Gardner).

No study has ever demonstrated the efficacy of artificially sweetened drinks for the control of weight. They do not work. They have also been proven to be a cause of cancer. So just say no to that option. (N Engl J Med 2012;367:1407-16, Ludwig DS)

The reason that they are not effective is because a person's caloric intake is not as important as what is happening to serum insulin. It is insulin that is the main cause of obesity no calorie intake.

Carbohydrates
Carbohydrates vary in their impact on insulin levels. High

glycemic index carbs produce more than twice the spike in blood glucose as low glycemic ones. This increased production of glucose also lasts for five hours instead of four. Dietary fiber tends to moderate the conversion of carbohydrates to glucose. This is why unrefined carbs produce a smaller increase in glucose and therefore less insulin production. One pound of mixed vegetables, nuts and berries has the same glycemic impact as one hamburger bun. Refining is the real problem as it removes the naturally occurring fiber and fats that slow down the conversion of the carbs into glucose.

Studies have shown that a diet high in fiber reduces insulin production in type two diabetics. (NEJM 342, May 11, 2000 1392-98). You should not consume a high fiber diet if you have had a heart attack as studies have shown it to produce a 25% increase in recurrent heart attacks. Fiber does not prevent colon cancer either but tomatoes and broccoli consumed together at least twice per week do. Coffee enemas will also prevent colon cancer as well as liver disease. Just so you know! (N Engl J Med, April 20, 2000 342:1156-1162)

Until recently the only thing food producers processed where carbohydrates but then they added processing and modification of dietary oils and then meats so now the entire food chain is involved. This is why junk food is so bad for you it is 100% processed and enhanced for preservation and flavorings. We must always try to eat real foods. Not edible food like substances.

Ray Reynolds

5 DIETARY SOLUTIONS FOR INSULIN RESISTANCE

In the last chapter we acquired a working knowledge of how high levels of insulin drive insulin resistance and excess fat storage. In this chapter we will examine the details of how to easily control these causes and loose fat as efficiently and effortlessly as possible. The following two pages of information concern themselves with the initial stage of the weight loss cycle. This is the initial loss of fat due to being in ketosis and using your fat stores for energy instead of blood sugar. The rate of loss is much faster than a calorie-restricted diet and more pleasant.

The second stage occurs after 4-6 months when your insulin production has dropped to normal levels and your metabolic thermostat starts functioning properly and burning off the remaining fat as body heat as fast as it can to return you to a 10% body fat level. Weight loss is so rapid that a difference in body fat is noticeable over a 24-48 hour period of time.

Eventually after about 2-3 months of this you will stop losing fat although it will seem that there is still some subcutaneous soft tissue where the fat was originally most heavily concentrated. These are the empty fat cells. They are like empty water bottles. They are empty of fat but still take up space. They will take up to a year to disappear because they must die a natural death from old age and not be replaced by new ones.

A very critical factor so far as fat loss is concerned is whether or not the new lower fat percentage can be maintained for an extended period of time. Numerous studies have shown that a high protein high fat diet is much easier to maintain in the long run then calorie restricted ones.

One randomized study in 2010 tested the durability of five different diets. The results showed that the only one that allowed the participants to maintain their new weight for six months or more was the high-fat, low-carbohydrate diet.

N Engl J Med Nov 28 2010 383 (22) 2102-2113 Larsen TM)

From what we have seen so far this type of diet is the only one that works for initial weight loss and is protective against regaining the weight once it is lost. It has also been proven to be more heart healthy than the low fat diets normally recommended.

The reason for this is that the high fat low glycemic index diets allow you to consume more total calories especially fats, which prevents the down regulation of your basal metabolism so that the extra calories are burned off to generate heat rather than being stored as fat. It prevents the resetting of your metabolic thermostat that we previously discussed.

All of the dietary research studies published in the last ten years are very consistent in their conclusions. They all favor the high fat low carb diet as being the most beneficial for both initial fat loss as well as continuing fat control for extended periods after the initial diet period. They are also healthier and more heart friendly than the other possible diet options.

No mater what type of diet you put people on there is always a 40% drop out rate. People always want to return to what they are familiar with and used to eating. Some universal conclusions that we can draw are:

1. All diets are difficult to follow.

2. Weight loss is much better on a high fat, low carb diet.

3. High fat, low carb diets prevent the down regulation of your basal metabolism.

4. A high fat diet does not increase you blood plasma LDL numbers enough to make a difference but does increase your good HDL cholesterol significantly. Also triglyceride levels are 30% better on high fat diets. Your body will produce its' own cholesterol to make up for any deficiency caused by diet. Cholesterol is the main ingredient in most of our hormones as well as making up 50% of our cell membranes and we will die if we do not have enough.

5. Consumption of fat does not make you fat.

There has been a steady rise in metabolic syndrome over the last 25 years, which is a precursor for heart disease. The symptoms are:

1. High abdominal fat percentage

2. High triglyceride levels.

3. Low HDL Cholesterol

4. Hypertension

5. High plasma glucose

Diets that are high in refined carbohydrates cause these same symptoms and that is the diet that we have been told to follow for the last forty years. The primary cause of metabolic syndrome is insulin resistance.

Consumption of triglycerides does not increase your bodies triglyceride levels no mater how much is consumed. Are you starting to notice that we can trust our bodies to sort out how much of various substances it needs to support its' processes? It will simply eliminate any excess it does not currently need.

Our bodies simply shut down their own production of whatever dietary substance that we consume in excess of its' needs. Fatty liver syndrome is actually caused by consumption of carbohydrates not fat. Fat accumulation in the liver is most often caused by carbohydrate induced insulin production, which causes fatty acid synthesis, which then accumulates in the liver.

The French produce fatty livers in geese by force-feeding them high carb corn mash. The result is called Foie Gras. If they force-fed them fat or protein this would not happen. Excessive refined carbohydrates are what give you a fatty liver not fat consumption.

Reducing your insulin resistance is not just beneficial for elimination of body fat and diabetes it is also a cure for metabolic syndrome all without the need for medications. Reduction of water retention is another benefit of insulin reduction. High levels of insulin cause our kidneys to retain water and salt, which causes edema or swelling of the ankles and calves. By reducing our levels of insulin we reduce the amount of work our hearts need to do as well. It reduces hypertension by lowering our blood volume.

Another problem with carbohydrate consumption is that because our genetics developed in an era when carbohydrates were very difficult to find we have never developed any limit to the amounts that we can eat. We cannot eat meat or vegetables to the point that it becomes unhealthy. But we have an insatiable appetite for cookies or ice cream.

Studies have proven that there is no satiation due to sugar consumption. It is very addictive. This is equally true of artificial sweeteners, which cause weight gain not loss. Our bodies closely regulate the consumption of unrefined carbohydrates so it is impossible for us to consume too much of them. Refined ones on the other hand are very addictive. A stack of pancakes with maple syrup will be consumed without stopping, green beans, not so much.

In studies of carbohydrate restricted diets it has been shown that once refined carbohydrate intake is stopped a person's caloric intake drops by as much as 1,000 calories per day. This is because the fats and proteins that are substituted for the high glycemic carbs are so much more filling.

Although the high glycemic index carbs are the main cause of insulin over production and resistance it has been found that all food groups including proteins and fats also raise insulin levels. A low carb diet is not a free ride either. They do not raise glucose levels but do raise insulin levels although obviously not nearly as much as carbs do.

Fats raise insulin levels the least of all the food groups. Proteins are however very effective at making us feel full for a longer time after eating. Dairy protein raises insulin levels the most and egg protein the least. Dairy protein should be avoided when possible in favor of eggs until your insulin is under control. If you drink coffee use cream which is 100% fat instead of whole milk. Also plant proteins produce much less insulin than animal proteins.

Hunger

Hunger is misunderstood. All it means is that your body is not getting enough energy. Two hormones that are secreted by the pancreas directly into the intestine cause the hunger sensation. They are Cholecystokinin and pancreatic peptide YY. Consumption of fat and protein makes us feel full. Which as we have noted is not the case with refined carbohydrates. Since our energy is being supplied by ketones when on a high fat diet we do not feel hungry.

Leptin

This hormone was discovered in 1994 and is released when we have eaten to make us feel full and stop eating. Your fat cells produce it so that the more fat you have the less hungry you feel. In a person with normal insulin levels this prevents over accumulation of fat. So the reasoning was that if we give people supplemental leptin it would make them lose fat. Unfortunately what they found was that the state of obesity is leptin resistant. Like every other hormone that is secreted in large quantities it is down regulated in fat people. That is one of the reasons that they are fat in the first place. So leptin supplementation only works for people with very low body fat who do not need it.

Cortisol

This is a separate cause of obesity. It is a product of stress. There is a direct correlation between cortisol level and abdominal fat. Sleep is also very important. There is a direct correlation between sleep depravation (less than 6 hours per night) and elevated blood glucose along with an elevated sensation of hunger. The reason for this is that the production of ghrelin is 28% greater when we are sleep-deprived. Lack of sleep also causes loss of muscle tissue. Observing the following rules will increase the probability that you will get sufficient sleep.

1. Sleep in complete darkness.
2. No TV or computer use one hour prior to sleep. The type of light they emit is the same as the sun and it causes the release of serotonin, which is what wakes us up in the morning.
3. 7-9 hours per night.
4. Keep your bedroom cool.
5. Have a regular sleeping and waking schedule
6. Loose fitting pajamas.
7. Older people may need to take 3 mgs of melatonin prior to

sleeping.

Take two tablespoons of Apple or Balsamic vinegar diluted in water after each meal and before going to bed. It slows down digestion and improves insulin sensitivity. It makes you feel more satiated. Vinegar also protects the heart. (NEJM Nov 25 2010 383(22) 2102-2113 Larsen TM)

Blood work numbers for high fat verses calorie restricted diet.

	High fat/Low Carb	Calorie Restricted
Body Fat % loss	-3.0	-01.5
Body Mass Index	-1.7	-0.75
HDL (mg/dl)	+5mg	0.0
Triglycerides (mg/dl)	-30	-15
Insulin reduction	-2.0	-0.2
Blood Glucose (mg/dl)	-2.0	-1.0
Systolic Blood Pressure	-7.5	-2.0
Diastolic Blood Pressure	-4.5	-1.0

All carbohydrates are made up of sugars. Simple carbohydrates are composed of one or two sugars, whereas complex carbohydrates consist of very long chains of sugar molecules, which require longer for our digestive systems to break down into their component simple sugars and utilize.

Examples of simple carbohydrates would be glucose, sucrose and fructose. Vegetables would be examples of Complex carbs.

The more fruit juice that a person consumes the higher their chance of becoming obese. This is especially true of commercial fruit juices that usually have sugar added. You need to institute a scorched earth policy of zero sugars or artificial sweeteners in your diet. That alone is usually enough to reset your insulin sensitivity over time.

A 1999 study of 50,000 women found that participants who drank more than one soft drink per day gained eight pounds of fat per year. Those who drank less than one per week only gained four pounds per year. Those who discontinued drinking all sweetened drinks did not gain any fat. The three things that are making you fat are Sugar, Sugar and Sugar. The probability of you developing diabetes is 80% greater if you drink more than one sweetened drink per day.

It is not the glucose that drives the obesity it is the insulin that drives it. The glucose is simply what causes the high insulin level. Your systemic level of glucose is determined by how quickly you digest carbohydrates. This is why complex carbs do not raise your glucose level as much.

It takes longer for your digestive system to unravel them into their component sugars so that there is a slower release over a longer time causing less overall insulin production. Fiber either as a part of the complex carb or dosed separately slows down our digestion as well. Vinegar also slows digestion causing slower release of glucose and therefore insulin.

Fructose is the sugar from fruit. It does not raise your blood glucose level. So you would think that you should be able to use it without increasing your insulin level. If your daily intake of fructose is provided by eating fruit you would only be able to ingest 25 grams of fructose no mater how much fruit you eat per day but if it comes from fruit juice you can very easily ingest more than 100 grams per day. That is based on your drinking only 100% natural juice that has no added sugar.

High fructose corn syrup
Sucrose (table sugar) is composed of 50% fructose and 50%

glucose. HFCS consists of 60% fructose and 40% glucose. Food producers love this stuff for the following reasons:

1. It extends the shelf life of products that it is used in.

2. It is cheaper.

3. It makes breads brown better when baking as well as keeping them soft.

4. It's sweeter than glucose.

5. It prevents freezer burn.

6. It is a liquid so it mixes faster and more completely than granulated sugars.

Because low fat foods were so popular the food producers removed all of the fat from all foods and put big "Fat free" labels on everything. The problem was that food did not taste very good without the fat so they put enough HFCS and artificial flavors into their processed foods to give them flavor. Over the last few years the quantity of HFCS that is used in processed foods has continually risen and it has recently been vilified as the unhealthiest of the sweetening agents.

The problem is that glucose is the only form of sugar that can be used by our cells to produce energy. Fructose must be metabolized in the liver in order to convert it to glucose so that it becomes bioavailable. Unfortunately it is broken down into triglycerides, which are a form of fat that then causes fatty liver disease. The conversion process is independent of the amount taken in to our bodies so that if you consume a gallon of HFCS your liver will convert every drop of it to fatty acids. It can cause an 80% increase in the triglyceride levels of normal healthy people causing liver damage within one month. There is a direct correlation between fructose intake and triglyceride levels. (N Hanes Study 1999-2006).

Good cholesterol (HDL) also decreases proportionately with the intake of sugars but HFCS causes LDL to go up as well. All of the important and beneficial numbers become four times worse after the intake of HFCS as opposed to glucose. Hypertension becomes worse as well. Stopping the consumption of all sweet beverages produces a 10% drop in blood pressure.

If you take in glucose your body will stop utilizing it when it has enough to supply current energy needs and only the excess will be converted to lipids for storage in the fat cells. Every drop of HFCS will be converted to lipids. This is why HFCS causes fatty liver disease. The other problem is that HFCS does not stimulate the release of ghrelin and leptin causing you to feel full.

Test subjects who were given 1,000 calories of HFCS in addition to their normal diet had a 25% increase in their insulin intolerance over subjects that received 1,000 extra calories of glucose. So consumption of HFCS is 25% more likely to cause diabetes as well as fatty liver disease. The consumption of HFCS causes a 25% increase in Hyperinsulinaemia over the same amount of glucose consumption. Your blood sugar does not go up but your insulin production does.

Moderate fructose consumption can cause the onset of diabetes in healthy people after only two months. HFCS is much worse than other sugars because it directly contributes to the increase of insulin production without the intermediary step of raising your blood glucose.

All sugar-sweetened beverages are addictive. You need a progressively higher dose to get the same satisfaction level this is particularly true of HFCS sweetened beverages. Breaking this addiction is very difficult. This also causes an increase in total caloric intake because you still feel hungry. This works very well for the food producers and the medical establishment as well because you end up giving them more of your money to feed or cure your addiction to eating. This is the opposite of natural foods that reduce your feeling of hunger the more you eat.

Wheat

The wheat we consume today is not the same as 100 years ago. It has been altered not by the modern process of GMO gene splicing but rather through selective cross pollination until it has become what is called dwarf wheat. This type of wheat produces three times as many kernels as the traditional einkorn wheat that has been grown for thousands of years.

Because the tall stalks could not support the weight of so many kernels they developed a type that is only 25% as tall as the original Einkorn strain. This dwarf wheat is much less expensive to grow than the traditional type and requires less fertilizer. The shorter stalks are less likely to be damaged by heavy rains as well. Yield per acre is much greater and it ripens much faster.

Let's take a look at the nutritional aspects and see if it is as good in that respect. Since 1843 the Broadbalk Wheat Experiment has been testing various characteristics of the yearly wheat crops. In 1960 the yield per acre went from three to seven tons per acre. Unfortunately the nutritional values decreased, especially the amounts of trace minerals such as iron.

Legally flour producers can remove up to 70% of the wheat germ and still label the resultant flour "Whole Wheat". This lengthens the shelf life of commercial bread considerably and the manufacturer can also sell the more valuable germ that they remove separately for a higher price. Quite often they will add molasses to commercial bread to darken it and make it look more like "whole wheat".

All that multi-grain means is that the product has several

different types of grains. I can guarantee you that all of them have been adulterated. Most of the germ, bran and fiber have been removed. At the very least make sure that you are buying whole grain flour not just "whole wheat" or buy your wheat kernels in 50 pound sacks and purchase a flour mill designed for home use and make your own flour and bread.

There is a big difference between the way that wheat was ground in the past and today. A hundred years ago wheat was ground by hand between stones and was fairly coarse. This slowed down its' digestion and allowed the glucose in it to be released more slowly keeping insulin levels low. Today the modern mills turn it into dust, which tends to digest very quickly and spike glucose levels. So the way that grains are processed can affect their glycemic index just as much as hybridization.

70% or more of flour is endoplasm (the white carbohydrate part). Endoplasm is composed of amylopectin. Amylopectin C is the least digestible and is found in legumes (Beans). Amylopectin B is much more easily digested and is found in bananas and potatoes. Amylopectin C is the type found in wheat and is the most easily digested. Wheat unfortunately is the carbohydrate most easily converted to glucose. Whole wheat bread has a glycemic index of 70. Glucose is 100 and a candy bar has a glycemic index of 50. That's right, your typical healthy whole wheat bread will produce a greater insulin spike than sweetened chocolate.

Gluten is one of the proteins contained in wheat. When it is digested it produces what are called exorphins, which have a similar effect as morphine. They can also cross the blood brain barrier. So it is very possible that wheat is addictive. When we consider what types of foods are considered "Comfort foods". We find that most of them contain wheat products.

Pancakes

Spaghetti and meatballs
Mac and cheese
Pies, Cakes
Mashed potatoes and gravy

So the difficulty is not in understanding the problem and the implementation of the solution. That is fairly easy. The main issue is that we have to beat this cycle of sugar and wheat consumption driving up our glucose levels, which then increases our systemic insulin level creating type two diabetes, fatty liver and metabolic syndrome.

This is only difficult because of the addictive nature of all high glycemic foods, which are at the root of the problem. Bread, wheat, milk and sugar did not exist until humans became agrarian about ten thousand years ago. That amount of time is a blink of the eye in evolutionary terms and our genetics have not had enough time to adjust to them. The more of them that you can eliminate from your diet the better off you will be.

6 INTERMITENT FASTING

Until recently fasting has been an integral part of our very nature and existence. From the first proto-humans two million years ago to the agricultural revolution ten thousand years ago and even after fasting has been a part of our lives. Granted it was not voluntary until more modern times but it didn't need to be. It was a fact of life that molded our genetics into what it is today and we ignore its power to cure us at the risk of our overall health.

If you want to produce a combination of despair and terror in a person try suggesting that they fast. This reaction is caused by the feelings of intense hunger they have felt when they missed a meal. What you need to understand is that once you start down the road to reducing your insulin levels it becomes progressively easier not to eat. If I am doing something interesting it may be four of five in the afternoon before I feel any hunger and decide to have an early dinner instead of a late lunch. This is called intermittent fasting and is basically the extension of the length of time between meals ultimately to the point where you skip one.

The world record for fasting is 382 days by a man who was placed on a fast by doctors so that he would loose weight. He felt so good on the fast that he remained on it until he had lost 276 pounds of fat and weighed only 180 pounds. He was monitored throughout the fast by physicians who reported no ill effects from his prolonged period without food so you will probably be able to make it an extra 6-8 hours between meals with no adverse effects on your health.

Even after a year his blood work was normal. His blood glucose levels were very low but acceptable and his mineral and electrolyte profiles were normal. The only abnormal parameter was that his insulin levels were very low, which is logical since he was running on ketones for most of that time and high levels of glucose were never present to trigger production of insulin. Also his growth hormone levels were elevated but that is a good thing.

As we saw earlier any type of caloric restriction causes our basal metabolic rate to slow down to conserve energy. This does not happen when we fast. That is illogical but true. What happens is that if you consume more than about 100 grams of carbohydrates per day your body will continue to try and use carbohydrates as your primary energy source.

If you discontinue eating carbohydrates completely your body switches over to 100% ketone utilization mode until such time as you disrupt it by eating carbohydrates. When that happens your body assumes that you have discovered a food source and switches back into glucose utilization mode. If you then consume less than say 2,400 calories per day it assumes that there is a food shortage and down regulates your basal metabolic rate to compensate.

Speed of transition from one to the other is the key factor. When we were hunter-gatherers we either had a very large supply of carbs (the apple tree) or none. We were either stuffed with high carb food and storing fat or we were wandering about looking for more of the same and burning our fat stores. It was one or the other not both at the same time. When we try to reduce our caloric intake to reduce fat but are still consuming more than 100 grams of carbs per day our bodies assume that we have found that apple tree and have only eaten a couple of the apples and that for some reason we have stopped eating them.

This is unacceptable and our bodies release more hunger hormone to inform us that we need to eat more to build up our fat stores. When that doesn't happen it starts shutting down our metabolism to conserve what it considers to be rapidly dwindling energy supplies. The end result is that when we are in ketosis we do not feel hunger unless we eat some carbohydrates and stimulate the hunger response for them.

Studies of alternate day fasting have shown that there is zero reduction of metabolic rate from being in a fasted state but the second that you eat a very small amount of carbs your body expects more and switches over to trying to use glucose for energy production.

The important thing for type two diabetics is that their insulin sensitivity doubles after only two weeks of alternate day fasting. It also doubles their adrenalin secretion, which greatly increases their energy level and alertness. This would be the equivalent of hunting mode for our ancient ancestors. Looking for that next meal we needed all of the energy and alertness possible to succeed.

People actually feel better fasted than when they are eating too much. The thing to remember about fasting is that your metabolism and energy use remain the same but you are using up fat to produce that energy not relying on the continuous intake of carbs to produce it. That is a win/win for fat loss.

The reason that more growth hormone is released during fasting is that it aids in the conversion of the fatty acids used when we are in ketosis. Growth hormones also promote healing of damaged tissue and general health. So there is really no logical reason to avoid being in a fasted condition.

If you are a chronic over eater particularly if you tend to binge eat it is probably being caused by insulin resistant hypoglycemia. This is when you increase your glucose levels but you're cells' receptors are so desensitized that no glucose is moved into them so more insulin is secreted until you reach a tipping point where too much glucose is removed from your blood and you do not have enough to supply your body's basic energy needs.

Your body does not have enough time to switch over to ketone production. This can result in confusion, dizziness and becoming unconscious. Normally you just become very hungry and eat anything you can find. If that something is very high carb your blood sugar will spike again resulting in another release of insulin and blood glucose depletion followed by another eating session.

The length of time between crashes and eating sessions will vary according to the glycemic level of the food you binged on. Five candy bars, about 45 minutes, a steak and green beans maybe never. Obviously fasting will cure this as well by eliminating the glucose/insulin rollercoaster and giving your insulin receptors time to normalize.

Since you are living off of ketones when on a high fat diet, the same as when fasted, metabolically they are almost the same. Fasting also results in a reduction of LDL cholesterol and triglycerides while maintaining your original HDL level.

There is a surgical procedure called stomach stapling that is used to cure obesity. Basically it reduces the size of the stomach to that of the intestine. 90% of the diabetics who undergo this procedure are cured of their diabetes. It is a form of forced fasting. So why not just do without the operation and fast. It will produce the same results.

Taking diabetic medications usually does not do anything for type two diabetics except worsen their condition. Fasting is bariatric surgery without the surgery. Another advantage to fasting is that it is easily reversible, just start eating again, Surgery unfortunately is not so easy to reverse. During WWII both sugar and flour were rationed and levels of both heart disease and diabetes plummeted.

7 DIETARY DISEASES

Although you are probably reading this book because you want to lose body fat that is really the least of the benefits of controlling your insulin production. Earlier we listed some of the diseases that are made worse by, if not directly caused by over production of insulin. They are:

Metabolic Syndrome
High Triglyceride levels
Hypertension
Fatty Liver
Diabetes

There is another group of diseases that are termed Western Diseases because they primarily exist in the US and Europe. They are:

Coronary Artery Disease
Obesity
Diabetes
Colorectal Cancer
Breast Cancer
Tooth Decay
Constipation

These diseases did not exist in primitive societies throughout the world until their diets came under the influence of the West. Up until the 1920s Native American people had an incidence of cancer and coronary disease that was almost zero. The same was true of the Eskimos of Alaska and Canada. Since that time these diseases have become progressively more prevalent in these Native North American societies.

The diets of these peoples were primarily fat and protein. This was also true of the Masai tribe of Africa and their immunity to disease, cancer in particular, was also well known. None of these cultures had any tradition of vegetable consumption. Our western medical establishment claims that eating meat will cause cancer and coronary disease and that we should eat more vegetables and less fat. This is the exact opposite of some of the healthiest people in the world.

At the other end of the dietary spectrum are the Tukisenta and Kitava Tribes who live in the highlands of New Guinea. Their diet is almost 100% carbohydrate. These people also enjoyed perfect health prior to the arrival of western civilization. No obesity, cancer of coronary disease. Other primitive tribes throughout the world enjoy the same great health even though their diets are 70-90% carbohydrate. Why are they neither obese nor diabetic? Studies conducted in the 1960s showed that the highest serum insulin levels of these primitive peoples was equal to the lowest levels in western societies.

(Metabolism, Vol 48, No 10, Oct 1999:1216-1219 Lindberg S)

The important lesson here is that it is not the carbohydrates that are causing the problem but the refining and concentration of them that creates the problem. I currently am living in Southern Peru where coca leaves are chewed to cure altitude sickness and provide energy. They work very well for both. If you take the same leaves and remove and refine the alkaloid they contain it becomes a white powder called cocaine which is not so good for your body.

Likewise the artificial concentration of most substances that we ingest is detrimental to our bodies. The basic rule of good health seems to be moderation in all things. Biology usually operates on moderation and pulsed delivery of any substance that it requires and not on the theory that if some is good then more is better. When considering any nutritional path always look at how our ancestors lived for advice. Most everything that they did will work just as well for us today.

What all of these various primitive societies have in common is that they do not eat any processed foods, refined wheat or sugar (the same as our ancestors in the Paleolithic).

Primitive Societies in transition

Tokelau Island is located near New Zealand and has been studied as it transitions from a traditional to a more modern culture. Their traditional diet primarily consisted of fish and coconuts (protein and fat). As they became more and more modernized their level of carbohydrate consumption increased.

In 1966 due to over population most of this island's people were moved from their island to New Zealand itself. Over a 15-year period from 1968-1983 their intake of sugar and flour increased dramatically from less than 2% of their caloric consumption to 15% causing an increase in weight of 20-30 pounds per individual. The incidence of gout, gum disease and tooth decay increased as well.

The native Maori of New Zealand are very fat despite being very active so apparently exercise is not much of a factor for fat loss. What is interesting is that in the 1800s prior to adopting a western diet the Maori were not fat. The rate of cancer has also doubled within these cultures after adopting diets high in refined carbohydrates.

Cancers are of two varieties; life style cancers such as colon, lung and breast cancers, which are associated with a persons diet, and traditional cancers, which are not predominantly influenced by diet. The incidence of life style cancers within the native Alaskan cultures has increased by 25% as they have adopted more modern high carb diets.

Studies have also been done that examine their rates of cancer according to the amount of westernization that has occurred within separate groups. It was found that the more westernized a segment of their population was the higher the cancer rate.

The incidence of breast cancer in the US is twice that of Japan and even more interesting is that Hong Kong has a high rate of breast cancer whereas on Mainland China it is almost zero. The difference is that the population of Hong Kong is very wealthy and can afford the bad habits that contribute to cancer. The mainland population on the other hand has to grow their own food and has a traditional diet.

If however you move these Mainland Chinese women to the US their children have a 60% greater chance of breast cancer even if both parents are ethnic Chinese. This is 100% true of any traditional culture. Whenever they are relocated from their traditional environment to the US their probability of cancer increases exponentially.

There is a 40% greater risk of cancer in type two diabetics being injected with insulin. This is probably due to systemic inflammation caused directly by the high levels of insulin and is another reason to lower our levels of natural insulin production. (CJ Currie Diabetologia 2009 52:1766-1777) (Gastroenterology Vol127, #4 Oct 2004 1044-1050)

The rate of heart attack for Japanese and Chinese is also much lower in their traditional cultures than in individuals who migrate to the US. This phenomenon has been studied extensively through the years and various theories advanced to explain it. The research data in this area indicates that the consumption of refined carbohydrates especially sugars is the primary cause. Sugar and insulin are both highly inflammatory as is the entire process of storing and using fat for energy.

As has been stated previously or bodies have never developed a signaling mechanism that will tell us when to stop eating refined carbohydrates. The result is that we always over consume them. Fat, protein and fiber slow down the digestive process, which slows the rate of absorption of any carbohydrates. This has the effect of reducing the relative glycemic index of any carbs that are present in the digestive tract.

When they are missing from our meal because we loaded up on high glycemic foods the absorption of the sugars from the carbs is much more rapid causing a proportionate increase in their glycemic index. The consumption of two tablespoons of unsweetened balsamic vinegar after a meal is very beneficial for slowing down digestion. So your mother was correct. Eating sweets will ruin your dinner not to mention your general health.

There is a very direct correlation between insulin production and heart disease. High levels of insulin are associated with a four times increase in heart problems. Up until five years ago physicians were treating diabetes with ever increasing doses of exogenous insulin because reduction of glucose was always the primary goal.

In 2008 during a study of type two diabetics, where glucose was very tightly controlled by the injection of large amounts of insulin it was found that although the glucose levels were kept very low there was a 20% higher death rate from heart attacks over that of the control group whose insulin was much more loosely controlled so that the researchers were forced to discontinue their study.

Since then there have been two other studies that have shown the same results. Injections of large amounts of insulin to control diabetes are not a good idea for type two diabetics. This is logical since unlike type one diabetes type two is caused by over production not under production of insulin. Insulin has also been proven to promote hardening of the arteries which is another factor for increased heart disease. High levels of insulin make all types of heart disease worse.

This is confirmed by a study in 2013 of the death rates of diabetics who control their diabetes with metformin a drug that directly reduces blood sugar instead of raising insulin levels. There is an 80% increase in the mortality rate for patients who use insulin for treatment over the ones using metformin. Further studies have since shown that adverse coronary reactions to insulin injections cause a 60-300% increase in heart attacks over other types of treatment.

From this it should be obvious that if you have type two diabetes, which by definition produces very high levels of systemic insulin you should do everything you can to lower it not just to cure the diabetes but to prevent other medical conditions that might prove just as fatal. There has never been a study that showed that insulin injection does not cause a high percentage of death due to heart disease. This is being driven by the creation of metabolic syndrome, which is caused by the over production of insulin in type two diabetics.

8 FAT PHOBIA

Since the official US government war on fat began in 1977, ostensibly to prevent obesity and heart disease, it has become increasingly obvious that consumption of saturated fat has very few negative consequences but its restriction from our diets does. One of the main reasons for restricting fat consumption was to lower cholesterol levels, which it was thought would decrease coronary diseases such as the formation of plaque on arterial walls.

Cholesterol is usually presented as a completely harmful substance that should be reduced as much as possible. The reality is that it is one of the most important and beneficial substances in our bodies. It is used in the manufacture of all of our hormones and it makes up 50% of a cell's membrane. A major component in the manufacture of cholesterol is saturated fat.

When the consumption of saturated fat is restricted our bodies are forced to substitute other types of fat for cell wall repair, which causes a decreased permeability and flexibility of those membranes. Cholesterol is so necessary for proper bodily function that every cell has the ability to make its' own.

For this reason restricting dietary intake of fats to lower our levels of cholesterol is futile since our bodies will simply make up for the shortage by producing its' own. As it turns out 80% of the cholesterol that we need is manufactured internally rather than being ingested. When we restrict our intake of cholesterol our bodies simple manufacture more to make up for the shortage.

In 1970 Ancel Keys published his study of fat consumption verses heart disease, which stated that there was a direct correlation between the amount of saturated fat consumed and the rate of heart disease. Because of this study the polyunsaturated and mono-saturated fats were declared to be the healthy alternatives to saturated fats. He started out with a sampling of 21 different countries, and then selected the seven that best exemplified his premise. It's called "Cherry Picking the Data" and is one of the most common forms of scientific fraud. He was very famous and well connected so his theory was accepted without supporting peer reviewed studies.

Vegetable oils were to be substituted for lard and butter. This then became the 1970-1980s war on saturated fats and cholesterol. The health authorities believed that by convincing the general public to stop consuming saturated fats they could eliminate heart disease within 15 years. The reality was that the US ended up with an enormous increase in diabetes, obesity, heart disease and metabolic syndrome.

Probably the largest and longest running study of heart disease was started in 1948 and involved the entire town of Framingham, Massachusetts. It is still ongoing and currently includes three generations of residents. While it is true that this study shows a small rise in death rate between the ages of 40-50, which is accompanied by a corresponding rise in cholesterol it is very small. When they looked at 60-70 year olds however the death rate leveled off and did not continue to increase with age even though their cholesterol levels increased.

What it shows is that as cholesterol levels increase they become protective and prevent death rather than cause it. While it may be true that very high levels of cholesterol can contribute to heart conditions it tends to be protective over all so far as longevity is concerned. There is actually an exponentially increased probability of death from general causes in persons with low cholesterol and in older individuals high cholesterol is very protective of over all health. This effect is greater in women than men. They are continuously protected by cholesterol no mater what their age.

https://www.framinghamheartstudy.org/

In a very recent study of 19 European countries that have very high cholesterol levels it was shown that their overall death rate from all health related causes was much lower than in countries with traditionally low levels.

The Framingham study has shown that there is a very wide variation in cholesterol levels within any community. Some of the residents have high levels and others low levels. Contrary to popular opinion this is not caused by variations in diet. That information is not normally made available but was published once on October 30th 1970

This study showed conclusively that people who consumed a large amount of fat had exactly the same cholesterol levels as those who consumed very little. The national Cholesterol education Program states that "Although high dietary cholesterol intake produces high cholesterol levels in lab studies of primates no such increase is found in humans.

So apparently there is no link between dietary fat consumption and heart disease. More recent studies have shown that overall life expectancy actually increases with high levels of dietary saturated fat consumption. What caused most of the confusion was that wealthier industrialized countries tend to have a higher percentage of heart disease compared to more pastoral ones. A part of the reason is that industrialized countries had switched to unsaturated vegetable fats, which have since been shown to cause heart disease not prevent it.

The Nurses health study of dietary fat and heart disease conducted by Harvard University studied 80,000 nurses over a 14-year period to determine which ones would get heart disease. This was the first study that conclusively demonstrated the link between heart disease and the consumption of trans-fats.

But what was more interesting was that it showed that there was no difference in the incidence of heart disease between those participants who consumed very large amounts of saturated fat and those who's consumption was very low. This same relationship applied when measuring consumption of cholesterol itself. The nurses who had very high levels of cholesterol consumption had no more incidents of heart disease than their colleges who had the lowest levels. A high glycemic diet however caused a 30% increase in heart risk. Saturated fats over all were shown to have a neutral risk of heart disease.

Out of eleven studies over the last 15 years not one has shown a correlation between saturated fat intake and heart disease. Also vegetable oils demonstrated no ability to protect against heart disease. One study of various diets found that people on the Mediterranean diet had a 30% lower incidence of heart disease. A vegetarian diet provides a 20% reduction. Consumption of nuts provides a 30% protection because of their high fat content (50%). Consuming a large amount of trans fats increases your risk by 30% rather than reducing it.

Saturated fats are fats in which every position in the fat molecule that can have a hydrogen atom has one. The molecule is "Saturated" with hydrogen. This causes them to be chemically stable and have a very long shelf life. For this reason food manufacturers have always preferred to use saturated fats in their products. When the tide of public opinion turned against the consumption of saturated fats the manufacturers created saturated vegetable fats by infusing them with hydrogen causing them to become stable so that they would not spoil and would have a long shelf life as well.

These were called trans fats. And you thought that trans fats were developed with your health in mind! They were solely for the convenience and profitability of the food processors. This is one of the main reasons not to eat processed foods. It is impossible to know what they will do next to increase their profits that will eventually be proven to be detrimental to your health.

Unfortunately they were very bad for your health. One of the problems with using vegetable fats is that unlike saturated animal fats they are very high in Omega-6 fatty acids. Animal fats contain a higher percentage of Omega-3 fatty acids, which are much more beneficial for health. The problem is that if a person consumes a lot of processed foods he is taking in a very high percentage of Omega-6 and this is very unhealthy especially for the heart. It is also very carcinogenic. Switching from saturated animal fats to polyunsaturated vegetable fats in the 1980s was one of the worst health policies ever implemented.

As a side note milk and meat in the US are full of hormones and additives and are best avoided when possible. Down here in South America, where I currently live, the meat animals are all pasture feed and no hormones are added. The cancer rate here in Peru is 50% less than in the US. In Bolivia it is 70% less. Their people cannot afford the bad habits that cause cancer. Cancer is a rich mans disease.

The health professional's study conducted by Harvard University in 1996 consisted of 43,000 subjects who were monitored over a period of six years. They were divided into five groups according to the amount of saturated fat that they normally consumed per day. The group that consumed the most saturated fat was 15% less likely to have heart related health problems than the group that consumed the least.

In a ten year study of 8,000 healthy Japanese men conducted in 1985 there was a 25% lower chance of stroke in the group who's diet was highest in fat compared to the group with the lowest consumption of fat. So it appears that a high fat diet is protective against heart attacks and stroke not the cause. Likewise the groups that had the highest daily intake of protein were less prone to strokes as well. There was also no correlation between the amount of salt consumed and incidence of stroke.

A more recent study published in the 1997 JAMA demonstrated similar results. The group that consumed the most dietary fat had a 5% rate of stroke whereas the group with the lowest fat consumption had a 15% chance of having a stroke. So the participants who avoided saturated fats had three times the probability of stroke compared to the group that consumed the most saturated animal fat. The researchers also found that the only category of fat that is not protective against heart attack and stroke are polyunsaturated and trans fats.

In 2005 the Swedish Malmo Center study of 29,000 men and women showed a direct correlation between the percentage of dietary fat and the incidence of heart disease. The more fat that the subjects consumed the less heart disease they had.

In the 1980s and earlier the standard French diet had the highest fat content in the world but they had the lowest rate of heart disease. Americans who consumed 60% less fat had a death rate from heart disease that was 60% higher. Now we know why. Studies have been done that correlate the diets of the different countries with their rates of coronary death. Without exception those countries with the highest dietary fat consumption have the lowest incidence of heart disease and death. Saturated animal fat is very protective against heart disease.

In 2009 Dr. Krause, head of the American Heart Association assembled the data from twenty different research studies conducted over the last fifty years to determine if there was any correlation between saturated fat intake and heart disease. This data showed that there had never been any proven correlation between high saturated fat consumption and coronary disease. Keep in mind that the AHA has always asserted that heart disease is caused by fat consumption but now apparently have finally reversed that position.

In a study of heart disease that used 58,000 Japanese men as subjects no correlation between increased saturated fat intake and heart disease was found. The subjects were divided into 5 groups according to the amount of saturated fat that they consumed. The ones who ate the greatest amount of fat had the lowers percentage of cardiovascular disease and stroke.

In another study of 400 women in 2004 that was reported in the American Journal of Nutrition the researchers divided the test subjects into five groups according to the amount and type of fat they consumed. They then performed angiograms of the coronary arteries to determine the precise amount or blockage that was present. Three years later another angiogram was done to determine any increase in the amounts of blockage between the groups.

Those who consumed very low amounts of saturated fat had the greatest increase in blockage. The group that consumed the greatest amount of saturated fat not only did not experience an increase in their coronary artery blockage after the three years but also had a decrease in blockage. Saturated fats actually seem to clean out rather than block arteries. The greatest increase in blockage occurred in the group that used polyunsaturated vegetable oils.

A study was reported in the April 1999 issue of JAMA that showed that people with a higher consumption of eggs have a lower incidence of heart disease. Egg yokes contain high levels of Taurine, which is necessary for proper heart function. Don't forget the side order of extra bacon! A 2013 study of eggs reported in the British journal of medicine shows no correlation between consumption of eggs and increased heart disease.

There have been at least six studies that have proven that nuts are very protective of heart health. Two Brazil nuts will provide the daily amount of selenium that your heart needs to function properly. People who consume a large amount of nuts each day have a 30-40% lower incidence of heart disease.

Omega 3 fatty acids

In Paleolithic times our dietary ratio of Omega-3 to Omega-6 fatty acids was 1 to 1. Today in the western diet it is as much as 1 to 30. This is primarily caused by the consumption of the vegetable oils used in processed foods, which have very high amounts of Omega-6.

This imbalance is a major contributor to both heart disease and cancer. Fifty percent of the daily caloric intake provided by a Western diet is made up of three foods; flour, sugar and vegetable oils. None of which provide any nutritional value but do cause cancer, obesity and heart disease.

A 2010 study of 4,000 participants showed that dairy fat is very protective against diabetes. The more dairy fat that is consumed the less the probability of becoming diabetic.

All of this is logical. For the last two million years our predecessors have acquired a large part of their energy from animal fat. If it had caused health problems that proved fatal then the process of natural selection would have eliminated that behavior at a genetic level.

So what happened back in the 1970s when all of these erroneous theories were first proposed? There was no objective testing of those original theories. It was an intellectual rather than a reality based analysis of the increase in coronary disease. The leading experts of the day who had the most political influence and hubris jumped to the wrong conclusion, which was then supported by the politicians and believed by the general public.

It was not until much later when these assertions did not seem be working out that sound research was conducted to try to find the objective truth. In recent years nutritionists and bio researchers have done real objective testing to either validate or disprove the original assertions. Whenever there is a contest between Nature and politicians put your money on Nature every time. She will win in the end. Just make sure that your own health does not become collateral damage in the ensuing battle!

Be aware that if you do not eliminate sugar from your diet and consume fats and excessive calcium at the same time the inflammation of your artery walls that is caused by your high blood glucose level and insulin production will cause plaque to form on your artery walls. The sugar consumption is what causes it not the fat and calcium consumption itself.

Statins

One anomaly in all of this is that cholesterol-lowering drugs such as Statins have been conclusively proven to protect us from heart attacks. However these drugs also affect five other biochemical cellular processes including lowering systemic inflammation. So their effectiveness may not be due to their reduction of cholesterol levels but to other factors. Also they work by blocking the internal production of cholesterol rather than reducing exogenous sources, which is not a good idea considering how vital the correct amount of cholesterol is for the maintenance of our cells.

9 NUTRITIONAL SUGGESTIONS

This chapter contains a few general health tips that will help your body cope with the transition to normal insulin production as well as improving your overall health.

Omega-6 to Omega-3 Ratio

An interesting clue to the obesity epidemic that is sweeping industrialized countries and the United States in particular, are the changes in Omega-6 to Omega-3 ratios in dairy, egg and meat products that are being consumed by their populations. Prior to the 1950s dairy cattle were pasture fed and cows gave birth in the spring when those pastures were especially rich in Omega-3 fatty acids. These Omega-3 fatty acids were then concentrated into the cow's milk. Omega-3 is also found in the eggs of free-range chickens that consume natural foods such as insects.

In the 1960s the demand for both eggs and milk accelerated rapidly with the result that farmers needed to find ways to exponentially increase the productivity of their chickens and cows. Not enough pastureland was available to maintain free range cows and chickens so factory farming was instituted whereby both cows and chickens were fed a diet of corn, soy and wheat. This resulted in eggs and milk that are very high in Omega-6 fatty acids. The end result is that our diets now contain an excess of Omega-6 fatty acids and almost no Omega-3. The imbalance is quite often more than 30:1 in favor of the Omega-6.

The correct ratio for proper health is 1:1. Omega-6 fatty acids stimulate the production of fat cells from the moment of our birth until we die. Omega-3 helps with the development of our nervous systems and increases the pliability of cell membranes while reducing inflammation and limiting the production of fat cells. Omega-3 is very protective against both heart disease and cancer. Make sure that all of the eggs you consume are from free-range chickens. The yolks will be a much darker shade of orange and they will taste better as well. Happy free-range chickens produce happy eggs with a much higher HDL profile.

The proper ratio of calcium to magnesium

The ideal ratio of calcium to magnesium seems to be about 2:1. In order to calculate your correct dosage of supplemental magnesium you will first need to determine your approximate daily intake of calcium. If you do not consume a significant amount of dairy products you can safely supplement 1000 mg of calcium and 500 mg of magnesium. However if you consume a large quantity of dairy products such as cheese and milk you will need to calculate the approximate calcium that you are receiving from them and subtract that from the 1000 mg of calcium supplementation.

The reason for this is that excessive calcium in our systems that is not utilized by biological processes can form kidney stones as well as plaque on the inside of our arteries. Dosages over 500 mg of magnesium on the other hand will usually cause diarrhea in most people. These parameters need to be tailored to the individual so you will have to experiment and come up with a ratio that seems to work best for you.

A proper level of magnesium is vital for the proper utilization of calcium as well as vitamin D by our bodies. Magnesium converts vitamin D into its active form at which point it can assist with the proper absorption of calcium into our bones. Magnesium also stimulates the production of the hormone calcitonin, which is utilized by our bodies to draw calcium deposits from our blood and soft tissues moving them back into our bones where they belong.

This lowers the probability of osteoporosis as well as arthritis, heart attack and the formation of kidney and gallstones. There is growing evidence that systemic inflammation of our vascular system is what actually causes cholesterol and calcium to form plaque on their interiors. So making sure that 100% of the calcium that we consume is properly utilized is essential not only for the health of our bones but our cardiovascular systems as well.

Magnesium Gluconate is much more readily absorbed by our heart muscle cells, which require large quantities of it for proper function so it would probably be best to use that particular type of magnesium. Insufficient magnesium in our diets also contributes to inflammation and oxidation. Potassium is important because it regulates proper heart rhythm, blood pressure, hydration, digestion and muscle cell contraction.

Best natural sources of vitamins and minerals

Vitamin A	1 Sweet Potato	550% of your DV
Vitamin B6	1 cup Chickpeas	55% of your DV
Vitamin B12	One Clam	1,400% of your DV
Vitamin C	One Bell Pepper	10% of your DV
Vitamin D	1 oz. Cod Liver Oil	140% of your DV
Vitamin E	One oz. Almonds	37% of your DV
Vitamin K	One cup Spinach	1,000% of your DV
Calcium	One cup plain Yogurt	42% of your DV
Folate	One cup Spinach	65% of your DV
Lycopene	One Tomato	300% of your DV
Lysine	Two Eggs	100% of your DV
Magnesium	One cup Spinach	550% of your DV
Niacin	One cup Peanuts	100% of your DV
Potassium	One Sweet Potato	100% of your DV
Riboflavin	3 oz. Liver	100% of your DV
Selenium	One Brazil nut	100% of your DV
Taurine	4 Eggs	100% of your DV
Zinc	3 oz. Beef	100% of your DV

10 SUMMERY

As we have learned in the first chapters of this book Ketogenic diets are the only ones that are effective for both fat lose and the regulation of insulin production. Because of the richness and caloric density of Ketogenic foods you will eat less often and consume a much smaller quantity at each meal. When we are in ketosis 50-70% of our calories should come from saturated fats as well as the medium chain triglycerides found in such foods as coconut oil and avocados.

This high concentration of beneficial fats and proteins instead of high glycemic carbohydrates in our diet makes it easier for our bodies to switch over to burning our stored fat when the food in our stomach has been consumed. I view the hard-core Ketogenic diet as a temporary diet that can be used to quickly lower insulin production. Over time this in turn allows our insulin receptors to once again function normally.

The real benefit of the high fat/low carb diet is that it will eventually recalibrate our metabolic thermostat. Once this occurs fat loss is very rapid and automatic regardless of how many calories we consume. The problem is that it may take as much as six months on a Ketogenic diet before this recalibration is complete. During that initial period you will still lose more fat than you ever have before and not be hungry while losing it. But nothing can prepare you for the rapidity of fat loss you will experience when your metabolic thermostat starts to function properly.

My first thought when it happened to me was "This can't be healthy!" I guarantee you will never feel cold again. Your percentage of body fat will be determined not by how much you eat but by your metabolic thermostat, which will maintain your body fat at about 10% for men and 15% for women by burning off any excess calories as body heat. When you have lost the excess fat you can switch to a more varied diet such as the Mediterranean.

A very simple and easy test of your progress is to skip breakfast every morning and see how long it is before you become hungry. When you get up in the morning you have already fasted for 12 hours and your goal might be to make it to 12:00 and break your fast by having lunch. When you have become used to that and do not become hungry by 12:00 you would then extend the time that you are fasted for another couple of hours. When you are finally hungry you can eat a late lunch.

Keep doing this until you are able to go for 24 hours without eating any food. You can drink all the water, coffee and tea you want. You can use cream in your coffee and Stevia for a sweetener if you like. This has to be a gradual process that might require months to achieve. A very important part of this is having work and pastimes that are sufficiently interesting that it holds your attention so that you are not continually obsessing about food.

The ability to fast for 24 hours without feeling hungry indicates that your insulin production and metabolism have normalized. Alternate day fasting will cause a 50% reduction in insulin resistance every two to three weeks and is one of the fastest ways to eliminate over production of insulin. During Ketogenesis you should have a higher energy level than normal because it increases adrenalin production. The real power of a Ketogenic diet is it makes it easier to transition back and forth between a fasted and fed state.

Mediterranean Diet

The Mediterranean diet is currently one of the most popular and with good reason. Greek and Turkish foods are amongst the most flavorful in the world. This is a great maintenance diet once you have lost your fat and normalized your production of insulin. Just don't use it as an excuse to pig out on pasta and increase your insulin resistance. Some of the benefits are:

1. Provides quick weight loss.
2. There are many high protein and fat dishes.
3. A small amount is very filling.
4. It helps maintain low blood sugar levels.
5. It is simple to prepare.
6. People with elevated levels of insulin tend to see reductions.

There is even a Ketogenic version that can be found here: www.advancedmediteranean.com

Intermittent Fasting

Intermittent fasting is a great tool for lowering insulin levels and loosing fat at the same time. It is very synergistic when combined with the Ketogenic diet. You eat dinner a couple of hours before going to bed. If you eat at 7:00 pm and go to bed at 10:00 pm for example you would wake at around 6:00 am. At this point you have been fasting for 11 hours and your goal is to not consume anything but water or tea until around 2:00 am in the afternoon.

At this point you will have fasted for 19 hours and you can then eat enough to just satisfy your immediate hunger so that you can make it to 7:00 pm for your next Ketogenic dinner a few hours prior to bedtime. Combining a Ketogenic diet with intermittent fasting is one of the quickest and most effective means of loosing fat, especially if you are getting regular exercise as well. The website www.leangains.com is the place to go for detailed information on this type of program.

Fat Cell Apoptosis (Cellular suicide)

If you follow the advice about Ketogenic dieting and intermittent fasting you will probably find that you initially lose a very large volume of fat but that when you have lost about two thirds of the fat you started out with you suddenly stopped losing the remaining 30%. There is a very simple and logical reason for this. At this point you have very little fat stored in the remaining fat cells. They are empty but like empty one-liter water bottles the cells still take up space. It is only possible to lose two thirds of your apparent fat volume by diet alone.

At this point you need to wait until your body decides that you no longer will need those empty fat cells for future fat storage. The problem is that your body is programed to expend as little energy as possible. Preemptively destroying all of those billions of empty fat cells would require the expenditure of a great deal of energy. Also because fat storage has played such an important role in our survival our bodies want to keep those cells available just in case they are eventually needed.

Our bodies consider them to be survival gear and will keep them much the same as a person lost in the desert will carry an empty water container in hope of finding a source of water to fill it. The end result is that our bodies take a wait and see approach and allow the fat cells to die of old age rather than taking an active role in eliminating them. This process can take as much as a year to complete.

A big problem with trying to lose fat around your waist is that your body wants to keep it not just as a source of energy but also to protect your vital internal organs from cold weather. Fat is excellent insulation so your body will first eliminate all fat from your appendages such as arms, legs and face before using the fat that is stored around your torso.

All of this can be very frustrating and cause you to give up and go back to eating the same as you did prior to losing the fat, which of course will cause you to gain all of the fat back again. This is why any form of diet change has to involve lifestyle and mental changes as well. It has to go all the way to the core of your being and not just be a superficial attempt at improving your figure. What you need to understand is that it is not a steady state and that your strategy and mind set need to change along with your current metabolic situation. Here are some tables of Ketogenic foods to use as a guide.

Proteins	Calories	Fats g	Net Carbs g	Protein g
Bacon, 1 oz	176	14	0	12
Steak, 1 oz	69	4	0	7.7
Beef, 1 oz	70	4.3	0	7.2
Chicken, white, 1 oz	49	1.3	0	8.8
Chicken, dark, 1 oz	58	2.8	0	7.8
Egg, 1 oz	46	3	0.25	4
Fish, 1 oz	20	0.1	0	4.3
Fish, Salmon, 1 oz	40	1.8	0	5.6
Ham, 1 oz	50	2.6	0	6.4
Hot dog, 1 oz	92	8.5	0.5	3.1
Lamb chop, 1 oz	39	0	7.3	6.0
Pork chop, 1 oz	65	4.1	0	6.7
Pork ribs, 1 oz	102	8.3	0	6.2
Scallops, 1 oz	31	0.2	1.5	5.8
Shrimp, 1 oz	28	0.1	0	6.8
Tuna, 1 oz	52	1.8	0	8.5
Turkey Breast, 1 oz	39	0.6	0	8.4
Veal, 1 oz	42	1	0	8

Vegetables	Calories	Fats g	Net Carbs g	Protein g
Asparagus 1 oz	6	0.1	0.6	0.7
Avocado, 1 oz	47	4.4	0.6	0.6
Broccoli, 1 oz	10	0.1	1.1	0.7
Carrots, 1 oz	10	0	1.5	0.01
Cauliflower, 1 oz	7	0.1	0.5	0.5
Celery, 1 oz	5	0	0.3	0.7
Cucumber, 1 oz	4	0	1	0.2
Garlic, 1 clove	4	0	1	0.2
Green beans, 1 oz	10	0.1	1.3	0.5
Mushrooms, 1 oz	6	0.2	0.6	0.9
Onion, white, 1 oz	11	0	2.1	0.3
Bell Pepper, 1 oz	6	0	0.8	0.2
Pickles, dill, 1 oz	3	0	0.4	0.2
lettuce, 1 oz	5	0.1	0.3	0.4
Shallots, 1 oz	20	0	3.9	0.7
Peas, 1 oz	24	0	2.8	1.5
Spinach, 1 oz	7	0.1	0.4	0.8
Squash, Acorn, 1 oz	16	0	2.9	0.3
Squash, 1 oz	11	0	2.1	0.3
Tomato, 1 oz	5	0	0.8	0.3

Diary Product	Calories	Fats g	Net Carbs g	Protein g
Buttermilk, 1 oz	18	0.9	1.4	0.9
Cheese, Blue, 1 oz	100	8.2	0.7	6.1
Cheese, Brie, 1 oz	95	7.9	0.1	5.9
Cheese, Cheddar, 1 oz	114	9.4	0.4	7.1
Cheese, Colby, 1 oz	110	9	0.7	6.7
Cheese, Cottage, 1 oz	24	0.7	1	3.3
Cheese, Cream, 1 oz	97	9.7	1.1	1.7
Cheese, Feta, 1 oz	75	6	1.2	4
Cheese, Monterey	106	8.6	0.2	7
Cheese, Mozzarella, 1	85	6.3	0.6	6.3
Cheese, Parmesan, 1	111	7.3	0.9	10.1
Cheese, Swiss, 1 oz	108	7.9	1.5	7.6
Cheese, Mascarpone, 1	130	13	1	1
Cream, half-n-half, 1	39	3.5	1.3	0.9
Cream, heavy, 1 oz	103	11	0.8	0.6
Cream, Sour, 1 oz	55	5.6	0.8	0.6
Milk, whole, 1 oz	19	1	1.5	1

Nuts and Seeds	Calories	Fats g	Net Carbs g	Protein g
Almonds, 1 oz	170	15	3	6
Brazil Nuts, 1 oz	186	19	1	4
Cashews, 1 oz	160	13	7	5
Chestnuts, 1 oz	55	0	13	0
Chia Seeds, 1 oz	131	10	0	7
Coconut, 1 oz	65	6	2	1
Flax Seeds, 1 oz	131	10	0	7
Hazelnuts, 1 oz	176	17	2	4
Macadamia Nuts, 1 oz	203	21	2	2
Peanuts, 1 oz	157	13	37	0
Pecans, 1 oz	190	20	1	3
Pine Nuts, 1 oz	189	20	3	4
Pistachios, 1 oz	158	13	56	0
Pumpkin Seeds, 1 oz	159	14	1	8
Sesame Seeds, 1 oz	160	14	4	5
Sunflower Seeds, 1 oz	150	11	4	3
Walnuts, 1 oz	185	18	2	4

Ketogenic Recipes

Here are some standard Keto recipes to get you started. They are mostly desserts and all of them taste like their high carb relatives but eating them will cause you to lose fat. You can find thousands more on the Internet. www.ruled.me is one of my favorite sites for recipes.

Avocado Mint Chocolate Chunk Ice Cream

I make 4 kilos at a time and freeze it in small containers.

Ingredients

Mint flavoring to taste (preferably natural white powdered mint)
Vanilla flavoring to taste (preferably natural powdered vanilla)
2 ripe avocados
1-cup coconut milk
Half-cup heavy cream
Half-cup of unsweetened baker's chocolate cut into 1/4" chunks.
Sweeten to taste with powdered stevia

Preparation

1. Cut the avocados in half and scoop their insides into a bowl.
2. Add the cup of coconut milk, half cup of heavy cream and 2 tsp. Vanilla.
3. Blend this mixture together until smooth and creamy.
4. Blend the chocolate chunks and stevia into the avocado mixture.
5. Put the bowl in the freezer for about 10 hours to freeze.
6. Remove from Freezer 40 minutes prior to eating so that it can soften.

Keto Maple Syrup

Ingredients

3/4 Cup of water

1 Tbsp. of unsalted butter

2 1/4 tsp. Coconut Oil

2 tsp. maple extract

1/2 tsp. vanilla Extract

1/4 tsp. xanthan gum to thicken

Sweeten to taste with stevia

Preparation

1. Mix your butter, coconut oil, and xanthan gum together in a microwave safe container.

2. Microwave the mixture for 40-50 seconds.

3. Mix microwaved oils and water together.

4. Add vanilla and maple extract and powdered stevia to taste. Thin with water if needed.

5. Microwave for 40-60 seconds, stir, and let cool.

Keto Pancakes

Ingredients

4 Tbsp. Heavy Cream

4 Tbsps. of flax seed

2 Eggs

2 Tbsps. Peanut Butter

2 Tbsps. Keto Maple Syrup

1/2 tsp. baking powder

1 Tbsp. Butter

Preparation

1. Mix Peanut Butter, Maple Syrup, and eggs together.

2. Add the 4 Tbsp. Heavy Cream.

3. Mix in the flax seed and baking powder.

4. Grease a pan with butter at medium heat.

5. Cook the pancakes until the tops bubble then flip over. Cook for an additional 1-2 minutes.

Strawberry Preserves

Ingredients
16 oz. Fresh Strawberries
Powdered Stevia
5 tbsp. Chia Seeds

Preparation
1. Slice the strawberries into small pieces.

2. Place strawberries in a pan over medium heat.

3. Let it boil for about 5 minutes, until the juice has thickened slightly.

4. Add the chia seeds and stir for about 2 minutes. Remove from heat and let cool. The Chia Seeds produce a coating of gel when in contact with liquid. They will thicken the jam and are very good for you as well.

Strawberry Milk Shake

Ingredients
1 cup Coconut Milk
1/2 cup Heavy Cream
1/4 cup Milk
4 tbsps. of the keto strawberry jam
2 tbsps. coconut oil
4 Ice Cubes

Preparation

Place the ingredients in a blender. Blend to the consistency you want. The strawberries will cause the milk to thicken so if you want a thicker shake add more strawberries and milk.

Keto Chocolate Chip Cookies (2g Net carbs per cookie)

Ingredients

1-1/2 cups Almond Flour
5 tbsp. powdered egg whites
3 tbsp. Coconut Flour
3 tbsp. Psyllium Husk
10 tbsp. Unsalted Butter
3 tsp. Vanilla Extract
1 tsp. Baking Powder
2 Eggs
1 bar Unsweetened Chocolate diced into small pieces.
Powdered Stevia.

Preparation

1. Mix dry ingredients together.
2. Beat warm butter with an electric mixer for 2 minutes.
3. Add the egg and vanilla to the butter and beat until combined.
4. Sift the dry ingredients over the wet ones and mix well.
5. Mix the chocolate chips into dough. Divide the dough into 22 equal pieces.
6. Roll dough into balls, place on a cookie sheet and flatten.
7. Preheat oven to 350F and Bake for 15 minutes.

Ketogenic BBQ pulled chicken breast

Ingredients

2 boneless skinless chicken breasts.

3 cups tomato sauce

6 finely chopped garlic cloves

1 finely chopped onion

9 tablespoons cider vinegar

3 tablespoons Worcestershire sauce

3 teaspoons paprika

2 teaspoons freshly ground black pepper

2 teaspoons chili powder

1 teaspoon celery seeds

Add Stevia to taste

Preparation

1. Mix ingredients, except chicken, in a small pot over medium heat until they come to a boil.

2. Add Stevia and vinegar for sweet sour taste.

3. Add the boneless skinless chicken breasts and let simmer about an hour until very tender.

4. Use a couple of forks to shred the chicken breasts.

Thai Sweet and Sour Cucumber and Onion Salad

Ingredients

4 Large Cucumbers, unpeeled and sliced

2 Red Onions, sliced

2 Cup White Vinegar

1 Cup water

Sweeten to taste with Powdered Stevia

Preparation

1. Prepare the cucumbers and onions. Place them in a Tupperware container that has a secure lid.

2. Add the other ingredients.

3. Add more vinegar to increase the sour flavor, more Stevia to increase the sweetness or water to reduce both. Let it marinate for a few hours in the refrigerator and serve. This is very good with any rich spicy foods such as curries. The vinegar also slows down digestion helping to prevent insulin spikes.